The

YOGA

PRESCRIPTION

The

YOGA

PRE-

SCRIP

-TION

A Chronic Illness Survival Guide

Cory Martin

WRITEOUT

Published by Write Out Publishing

Published in the United States by Write Out Publishing,
California
www.writeoutpublishing.com

Some names have been changed
to protect the privacy of the individuals involved.

Interior Design by The Book Designers

Library of Congress Control Number: 2021941397

ISBN 978-0-9969193-3-3 paperback
ISBN 978-0-9969193-4-0 ebook

Printed in the United States of America

1 3 5 7 9 10 8 6 4 2

First Edition

To anyone struggling
with their "new normal."

CONTENTS

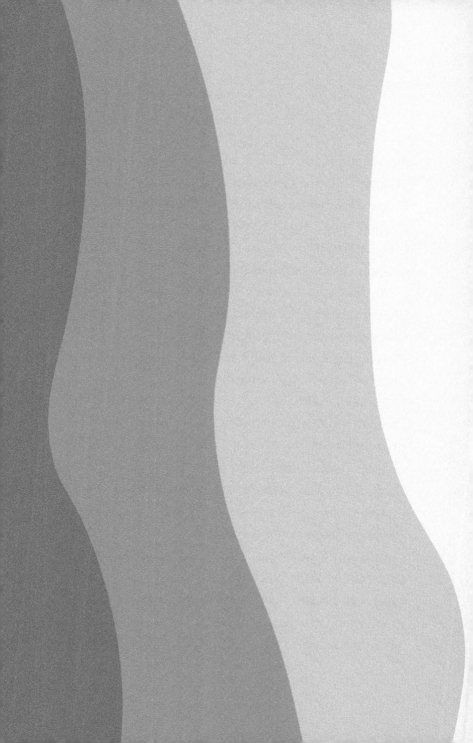

INTRODUCTION

I'm just going to come right out and say it: Dealing with a chronic illness sucks. All the doctors' appointments, the endless tests, the pain, the never knowing when and if your symptoms will get better or worse—it's a lot to handle.

I deal with multiple sclerosis and lupus. I've been on a roller coaster of health for over ten years now, and the only thing I know to be certain is that nothing is certain. Though I might be doing great today, tomorrow could be a whole different story. Some days I can walk five miles, others I can barely rise out of bed. I'm sure you can relate.

Luckily, I have something that keeps me sane in this crazy world of disease. Yoga.

I started practicing yoga in 2006, far before my health became chronic and painfully annoying. Yoga to me then was just an exercise class. I was 26 years old and carrying about 20 pounds more than my 5-foot, 4-inch body could handle. Since yoga had become synonymous with Madonna's ripped arms at the time, I took up the practice to get fit.

I arrived at my first class raring to go, but I was completely lost and terrified. I didn't know what I was doing. I had always been strong and athletic, but this required a strength I no longer possessed. My thighs quivered, sweat dripped down my brow, I was sore for days after—and yet, I left feeling amazing. That incredible feeling is what kept me coming back day after day. And it's what started to change me. Sure, my body dropped that extra weight and I became more toned. But more than that, I noticed I started to present myself differently. I had a newfound sense of confidence. I moved with ease. I was on a high. That same high, though it's not derived directly from the poses anymore, is what has buoyed me through my two diagnoses and the pain and fatigue that goes along with them.

There's a common misperception in the Western world that yoga is only the poses, or asanas. But yoga is far more than that. Yoga isn't a magic pill or a cure-all. Instead, yoga is another piece you can add to your treatment plan. When I talk about yoga now, I talk about it in the same way I talk about the drugs I take to manage my diseases—it doesn't fully cure me, but it helps me cope with the world around me. Yoga is a practice that evolves as you evolve—day to day, month to month, year to year, diagnosis after diagnosis, symptom after symptom. When I feel defeated, yoga picks me back up. When I am drained by my daily activities, yoga replenishes me. When I can't get out of my head and stop worrying about my future with disease, yoga helps me clear my mind. When my body fails me in all its symptomatic ways, yoga becomes my guide.

Regardless of what you may be suffering from, it can be your guide, too.

Yoga is not restricted to the healthy, the lithe, and the spry. Yoga is for every body. Wherever you are with your illness, you can do yoga. If you're stuck in bed for the day, week, or month, or use assistive devices, or fully mobile: All of yoga is accessible to you.

This is not your typical yoga book. It is not a prescriptive, *do this and you'll feel that* kind of book. Instead it's the kind of book that provides guidance to help you reach a place of feeling good, or even simply better. While this book does include the how-to of a variety of poses, they are not the focus. The real work and the real focus are on how to use those poses to access and live the philosophies of yoga to navigate life with chronic illness. I have been practicing yoga for over 15 years and teaching for almost 10. All the knowledge I have and will share with you is information I've learned along the way—as a student, a teacher, and a patient. I provide tales from the front lines of living with illness to show how I use yoga to cope. I break down the philosophies into digestible bits of information and reveal how yoga can become part of your life in a practical way.

Because I deal with MS and lupus, most of the book will be referencing those diseases, but please know that this practice can be adapted for any condition—chronic pain, rheumatoid arthritis, ulcerative colitis, fibromyalgia, ME/CFS, cancer, stroke, diabetes, and more. You can take away pieces from every bit of this book and cultivate your own yoga practice to match who you are in this very moment.

I often tell my students not to worry what the person next to them is doing. We are all on a different path. This is also true when it comes to our health. We all face our own illnesses, and deal with them in the best way we know how. Wherever you are in life, embrace the fact that you're here right now; and in this moment you are about to take a big step forward on this journey we call a yoga practice. Enjoy the journey and don't worry about the outcome, simply embrace the learning process.

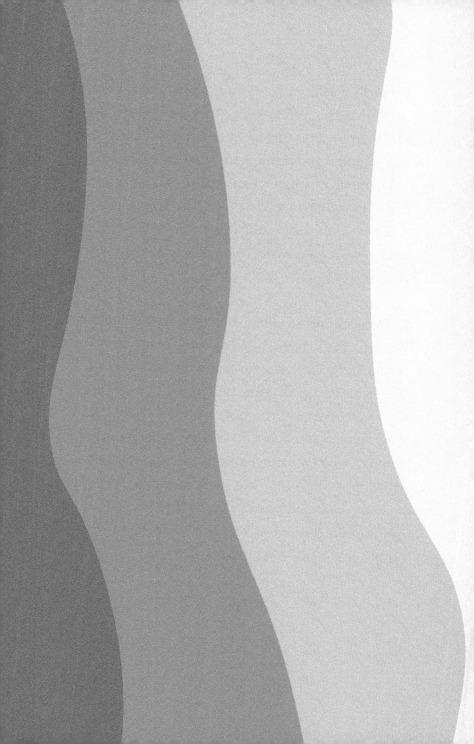

CHAPTER **ONE**

The Diagnosis

Every one of us has a diagnosis story. Sometimes it encompassed years of our lives as we struggled to find answers to troubling symptoms. Sometimes it arrived seemingly overnight. Sometimes we had other thoughts on how our lives would unfold, but then the diagnosis was given and everything transformed. The day we were told our lives would forever be changed is a day we will never forget. We might not remember the exact words of our doctor, but we remember exactly how we felt.

When I was 26 years old and had just begun practicing yoga, I thought I knew how my life story would unfold. It would be simple. Girl goes on a mission to get in shape. Girl does yoga. Girl gets fit. Girl succeeds in her career. Girl finds love and happiness. The End. But the get-in-shape part was really just the beginning of a far more complicated story.

In the fall of 2007, after a year of practicing on my mat, I thought I had finally reached that yogic state everyone talked about. I was calm, happy, and I could fit back into my skinny jeans. I thought I was totally enlightened. Okay, not really, because the jeans were Levi's and everyone knows that enlightenment comes from True Religion, but all was good—well, except for one thing.

I couldn't sleep.

At first, I ignored it. I told myself insomnia happens to people all the time. There was no need to be alarmed. I just had a creative mind that never shut down. But the truth was, it had nothing to do with my head and everything to do with my body. Something was not right. As hokey as it sounds, after doing so much yoga, I was very in tune with how my body worked, and this new state was not its normal state of operation.

In the middle of every night I would awake in pain. My arms, neck, and upper back were completely numb, and it took minutes, sometimes hours, for any feeling to return. For a while, I blamed the numbness on a weird sleeping position, but when I started to forget simple things, or things I had known forever, I decided to tell my doctor. During a routine physical I mentioned the lack of sleep, numbness, pain, and forgetfulness. I expected her to give a simple explanation like I needed to eat more carrots, or exercise more, but she was concerned. "This is not normal," she said.

She sent me to a neurologist who poked and prodded and tested my reflexes. I was completely freaked out. *Could something serious be wrong with me?* The neurologist immediately saw that something was off with one reflex, so she drew vial after vial of blood and sent me for an MRI of my brain. After months of tests and waiting around for results, the neurologist finally had some answers.

"I believe you have multiple sclerosis," she said.

"Are you sure?" I exclaimed. I had googled my symptoms before I had gone through all the tests. MS was a possible explanation but I didn't believe it could happen to me.

"I can start you on a drug now or you can see a specialist and get a second opinion," she said.

I chose the specialist, not because I thought she was completely wrong, but because in that moment I didn't want her diagnosis to be true. I wanted to put off my reality. A reality that took me from being a completely happy 27-year-old girl who had discovered this cool new workout fad called yoga, to being told there were five lesions on her brain and the only explanation for them was multiple sclerosis, an incurable and potentially disabling disease.

I left the office in shock. Multiple sclerosis? The answer I received was not what I'd expected. When I returned home, I dissolved onto the floor of my apartment in tears.

Multiple sclerosis. Multiple sclerosis. The words of the neurologist echoed in my head, over and over. I clenched my fists and pounded the carpet. I curled up into a ball on the floor. I did what I could to make it go away, but it wouldn't leave. I wanted to hurt someone or something. I was pissed and I was in a spiritual state called: *Whatthefuckishappeningtomeisthisshitforreal?*

I cried out into my empty living room. My sobs were incomprehensible, but my heart was translating. Yoga wasn't supposed to lead me here. I was supposed to get happy. I was supposed to get in shape. I was supposed to have a great career. Instead, I'd been screwed by Sanskrit. The truth hadn't set me free, it had only brought me bad news.

I most likely had multiple sclerosis and it was very possible that one day I would wake up and no longer be able to walk.

The thought itself was paralyzing.

Any strength I had built over the past year through yoga seemed to disappear. I was on my floor in a pile of nothing. My breath was short and heavy. My lungs could barely move, crushed by anxiety and fear of the unknown. All I focused on was my future and all of the "what ifs?"

What if I had to use a wheelchair? What if my memory worsened? What if I lost control of my bladder? What if I could no longer see? What if? What if?

In the weeks that followed, I looked for answers on the internet—which was a mistake. Google only presented the worst-case scenarios. There were so many possible symptoms and things that could happen to me. I was worried, scared, and only focused on the negative.

In the months following the diagnosis, I began to live in constant fear that my body was going to fail me and I hated everyone who looked so blissful and strong in their bodies. I looked at others and wanted to be like them. I wanted to run down the street and not think: *This may be the last time I do this.* I wanted to focus on my work and not worry: *Will I have to go on disability one day?*

I wanted the doctor to take back what she said. I wanted to be healthy. I wanted to return to that ignorant state before I ever heard the words *multiple sclerosis*. I wanted to stop feeling like I was out of control. But I couldn't.

For a year in my yoga classes, I had been listening to teachers tell me not to worry about what other people could do on their mats. That we were all different and the point of the practice wasn't to covet what someone else had, but to celebrate our own individual strengths. I had gotten good at this. When I bent forward, it didn't matter that my fingers barely grazed my toes and the girl next to me had her palms flat on the floor. I knew that one day I would get there (and I did). I was happy that I could balance on my hands with my feet in the air, but didn't feel like I needed to show off to anyone. I was allowed to be me and everyone else was allowed to be them. We were all different and that was okay. But that day in the neurologist's office my perspective changed.

Everything yoga taught me flew right out of the window.

I grew jealous of everyone who was healthy. I got angry when I saw people who had made themselves sick because they couldn't take the time to take care of their bodies. I couldn't watch *The Biggest Loser* and listen to doctors tell the contestants they had given themselves type 2 diabetes and high blood pressure. I got mad at people who took the elevator in my apartment complex when they could just as easily walk up one flight of stairs. I got upset when friends complained of being fat when they had recently become pregnant. I wanted to shout at them, "Your body gets to do an amazing thing right now, enjoy it! Who cares about gaining 30 pounds?"

I was spiraling with hate and resentment. Despite the fact that I could still physically do everything I had done before my doctor gave me the news, my emotional state had completely changed. I was filled with rage. I was angry and mad and certainly not zen. I hated that yoga had forced me to see that something was wrong with my health, yet I still loved the practice. Ironically, the only thing that made me feel normal during this time was yoga. When I stepped into the studio, I forgot about the devastating diagnosis. I stopped thinking about living with a possibly debilitating disease. Instead, I focused on what I could do in that moment. I rejoiced in the fact that I could breathe. I was happy that I could still stand and balance on one leg. I found joy in the sweat moving across my brow.

So I kept going to class and eventually, my practice shifted from a superficial *I want to look good* kind of practice to one that fully transformed my relationship with my body, my mind, and my disease.

At the beginning of a yoga class, the teacher often asks you to set an intention. My intention during the time of my MS diagnosis was always: *My body is a powerhouse.* Though I knew that my body could fail me at any moment, I also knew that my mind was an incredibly powerful thing and if I told myself that I was physically able, that I was indeed a powerhouse, then maybe I could remain powerful... And I did.

For ten years, the multiple sclerosis remained at bay. I experienced small bouts of fatigue, some difficulty in finding the right words (what they call cognitive fog), and the occasional MS hug—a girdle like sensation around the ribs that makes it difficult and painful to breathe. Other than that, I was living a healthy, normal life.

My writing career was back on track. I became a 500-hour certified yoga teacher. I taught in studios with some of the world's most renowned teachers. I taught private lessons to classes of one, and on the Santa Monica Pier to classes of hundreds. Everything was going well. I was happy and content and my physical well-being was great. The original life story I had in mind was coming true. But then, at the age of 38, my body started to fail me again.

I thought it was the MS finally coming to take hold. I battled fatigue that worsened day by day. I started to have deep bone pains in my legs and arms as if the growing pains of childhood had merged with the pains of exhaustion from being on your feet for 12 hours. I struggled breathing walking up three stairs. I got dizzy when I worked out. I lost the energy to complete the exercises I could do so easily a month before.

The MS doctor, however, was skeptical of my new symptoms. She didn't think they were MS. Three months of worsening symptoms and many other doctors and tests later, she was right. I was finally sent to a rheumatologist who assured me that he would get to the bottom of my pain. He would find out what was wrong, and he did.

"You have lupus," he said after reviewing the results of an extensive round of blood tests.

I sat in the chair across from him in a silent state of: *Isthisreallyhappeningtomeagain?*

How could it be lupus? Another incurable, unpredictable, life-altering disease.

"Are you sure?" I asked.

"Yes," he said. I waited for him to offer an alternate reality, but there wasn't one. This was real.

After living and adjusting to life with MS for so long, I thought I had seen the worst of what life could throw at me, but this felt worse. I was shocked speechless. I was lost. In pain. Fatigued. And I didn't know what to do.

I was put on a drug to control the inflammation in my body. Luckily, it worked. After a few weeks, some of the pain subsided. I had a little more energy, and could focus again. But I knew my life would never be the same again. My "normal" had shifted once more, so my practice had to as well.

I was physically unable to do much at all—taking a shower was exhausting. There was no way I could make it through an entire yoga class, but I also knew that if I didn't take care of myself, the lupus would take complete control of my life. I wasn't ready to give up. I needed a plan.

My doctors had their plan—driven by science, backed by studies and experience. They would prescribe meds as needed, monitor my health with frequent visits and blood draws, and help me manage my symptoms. This was all well and good, but I knew that I needed more than medical help. I needed a holistic approach to navigate my new normal. I needed a guide to help me survive and thrive. To do that, I leaned into the one thing I had spent over 15 years on, the one thing that grounded me and made me feel better: yoga. I looked to yoga to provide the framework for my new plan.

I began to explore how everything I'd learned over the years could help me through one of the most difficult times in my life. I went back to the philosophies, I took note of what poses felt right in my body, and which ones felt terrible. I observed the thoughts that ran on repeat in my mind and acknowledged that there were others I was avoiding. I became a graduate student of my health, devising a thesis and a strategy to deal with what lay ahead. I created my own treatment plan with yoga, tailored to my body's needs. My plan was full of trial and error and, like any good treatment plan, is still evolving. Even so, it is also my life force.

Yoga can be that for you, too. A powerful guide to help you feel good in your body despite your diagnosis. Yoga will help you survive, not in the literal sense, but in the sense that it will keep you thriving through the worst and best parts. It will provide a new perspective to living with illness.

Your yoga plan will be your yoga plan. It will not look like mine, your neighbor's, or others' reading this book. It will be unique to your body, your needs, your mental and physical states. Like anything worth anything, it will require work, but it will be the kind of work that will excite you every day. This yoga prescription will ask you to take personal responsibility for your well-being and it will be your best investment in yourself. No matter what you are dealing with you will be able to adapt this new treatment plan to fit your needs.

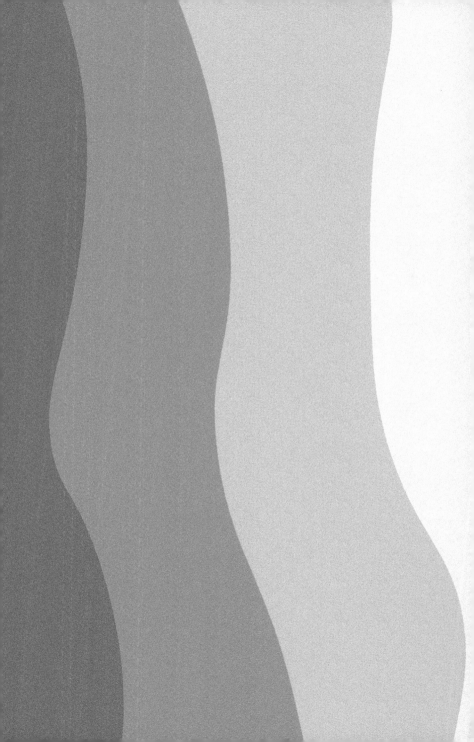

CHAPTER TWO

Understanding the Treatment Plan

After every diagnosis, there is always a proposed way to treat the disease. Sometimes it's scary, sometimes it's a godsend, sometimes you have to wait for insurance approval. But no matter what, you always have to understand the treatment plan. There isn't a drug I've been prescribed that I haven't read the full pamphlet to understand all the possible side effects and weighed the pros and cons. Sometimes I go so far as to research the mechanisms by which the drug works. I definitely don't walk in blindly, and neither should you. Hence the notion here: Before you begin your treatment plan with yoga, you must understand what yoga is.

WHAT IS YOGA?

Put simply, *yoga* means to yoke or bring together. It is the union of the body and the mind. In the same way that many medical practices are shifting their focus to the entire body—not just the "sick" part—to treat illness, yoga is meant to address your entire being. There is no yoga for the ankle. There is no yoga for the brainstem. Sure, there are poses that may strengthen or lengthen the muscles around your ankle and there are great meditations to enhance your brain, but yoga isn't just about focusing on one part of the body and making it well again. Yoga is about bringing your body and mind together to work in synchronicity.

As someone who lives with chronic illness, you probably already know that your body and mind are equally influential on how you feel day to day. When I'm in excruciating pain, it affects my mind. I become depressed, withdrawn, angry. The same is true in reverse. When I'm depressed, stressed, or anxious, my physical body is affected. My heart races, my breath becomes shallow, my muscles tense. At times, this can become a vicious cycle. When everything hurts, I don't want to move, and when I can't move, everything upsets me. And because I'm not stretching or moving my body, my body becomes stagnant and tight, which hurts even more, making me even more upset. This is the bad cycle.

On the other hand, if I wake up in the morning with energy and no physical pain, I see the world in a different light because I'm just so happy. When my mood is elevated, I want to keep moving, even if it's only a short walk around the block. And because my body's moving, I keep feeling better and better emotionally. This is the good cycle.

The good cycle is my holy grail. If I can get the good cycle to perpetuate for any amount of time, then I'm in a better place overall. Unfortunately, since I live in the world of unpredictable illness, I will always move in and out of the good and bad cycles.

The goal then is to diminish the length of the bad cycles. The goal is to figure out a way to keep knocking myself out of that vicious cycle of pain and anger and back into that bright cycle of energy and happiness. Since there is no cure for either of my illnesses, yoga became the answer to managing my new "normal."

Yoga taught me to rise again after getting knocked down. In the same way I might lose my balance and get right back up, the tools of yoga—its philosophies and teachings—teach me that no matter how often I fall into the bad cycle, I can always get back to the good. It can do the same for you.

YOGA'S TOOLS

At its core, yoga is the union of the body and the mind, but yoga also emphasizes the here and the now—the present moment. This *be present* philosophy of yoga is derived from a work called the *Yoga Sutras.*

Sometime around the first or second century CE, a man named Patanjali wrote the *Yoga Sutras.* This body of work consists of 196 *sutras*, or stanzas, that explain the philosophy of yoga. That philosophy provides the tools to help you ride out the bad cycles and return to the good.

The first sutra can be translated as "Yoga is now." According to Patanjali's work, if you can constantly live in the now, meaning you don't fret about the past or worry about the future, you don't need any of the other sutras. However, chances are this is not you, or me, or the person next to you. If you live on this planet, living in the present is a challenging task. Add chronic illness to that equation and you probably find yourself really struggling. If you're like me, before you were sick living in the now was difficult. Now, it sometimes feels impossible.

There are days where I long for the past. I wish for the times when I could compete in triathlons, or teach spinning, or hike an awesome hike and look out over the Pacific Ocean, or ski that double black diamond in the Rockies in two feet of powder and not feel like I was about to pass out and die. Then there are days when I worry so much about my future that I don't even want to do anything. Why work today when it feels like there's no reason to keep pushing forward? I constantly flit from past to future.

Being in the now is hard, especially when we have to deal with so many unknowns on a daily basis. But the good news is there are things we can do to help us be present. Patanjali wrote the sutras because he understood that while the ultimate goal of yoga is to live in the now, he knew how difficult this is to achieve. Each subsequent sutra provides a way to reach the now. To help people in their quest to find the now, Patanjali laid out a path to yoga called *ashtanga*. This path consists of eight "limbs," the facets of yoga that we can use to help us in our daily lives.

They are:

Yamas – ways to find self-control
Niyamas – ways to find discipline
Asana – the physical poses
Pranayama – breath work
Pratyahara – learning to withdraw from the senses
Dharana – learning to concentrate
Dhyana – meditation
Samadhi – freedom from the mind and the body, which really means enlightenment

These eight limbs are what compose an entire yoga practice. As you can see, the poses, or asanas, are just one limb. Despite the fact that most people who talk about yoga put all the emphasis on the poses, there are seven other components to the practice that have helped me far more than touching my toes ever did.

Before we get into all of the limbs of yoga, I want to focus on the yamas and the niyamas. These are two of the most practical limbs to study for learning how to apply yoga to life with chronic illness. I like to think of them as the ten commandments of the yogic world—guidelines to follow to live a healthy and enriched life.

The *yamas* (ways to find self-control) are the non-tangible principles to live by, and the *niyamas* (ways to find discipline) are the actions we can take to move toward a more enlightened state. When I say "enlightened," I do not mean some weird hippy state that's reserved for spiritual beings. To me, "enlightened" means a state where I am content with where I am in life, but also self-aware enough to continue to make changes to improve my entire being. However you decide to interpret "enlightened" is the correct way to view these limbs of ashtanga.

YAMAS

Each yama has its own translation and philosophy, which I will explain. The yamas are:

> Ahimsa – non-harm
> Satya – honesty
> Asteya – non-stealing
> Brahmacharya – abstinence
> Aparigraha – non-greed

AHIMSA

Ahimsa means to do no harm. Many yogis often translate "do no harm" into life as being vegetarian. They believe that harming animals is off the table, which is great. I love puppies and I've been a vegetarian for years at a time, but for us living the chronically sick life, ahimsa takes on a whole new meaning. I apply ahimsa to my body and my health. I have no intention of putting my body through anything that will do it harm. Sometimes this means skipping a glass of wine or skipping a workout to rest in bed. Sometimes I have to question the drugs I'm recommended and weigh their side effects thoughtfully. I have to constantly be aware that the things that harm my body are innocuous to healthy people and I can't try to compare and keep up. Ultimately, I have to listen to what my body needs in order to do no harm.

SATYA

Satya is all about honesty. As your kindergarten teacher probably told you, honesty is the best policy. Honesty when you're dealing with illness means you stop faking it. If you're having a bad day, it's okay to admit it. If you're having a bad week, don't try to ignore things and push through. Ask for help. Take time off work. If someone asks how you're doing, you don't always have to say you're fine. Be honest with yourself and those around you. This might take some time. It took me nine months after my lupus diagnosis to finally be completely honest with my fiancé. He would always ask how I was feeling and often I'd say okay even if I wasn't. Now I can say, "I don't have the energy to shower, get ready, and go out to dinner. Can we order in?" Now I can be honest and tell him that I'm scared to take that awesome trip we planned because I'm worried about flaring up. Now I can ask for help when I don't have the strength to pull my weight with the household chores. I can practice satya and be honest with him.

ASTEYA

Asteya means to not steal. Yes, you shall not steal from another, that's a given. But here, it goes deeper. Asteya in our world means not stealing our precious energy from one day to the next, or stealing time away from the things that bring us happiness. Asteya reminds me of the spoon theory, which posits that we all wake up each morning with a certain number of spoons and each activity we do requires a specific number of spoons. When we run out of spoons, that's it, there's no energy left to do anything else in the day. Asteya means we should stop stealing from ourselves. We should not steal any spoons from ourselves just to appear "fine." This is a lesson I learned the hard way. Six months after my lupus diagnosis, I wanted so badly to enjoy every moment of a three-day concert with friends that I ignored all signs of my body telling me to slow down. I didn't want to miss out on a thing, and I didn't want to be the "sick friend" holding everyone else back, so I powered through and used every spoon I could find. After that weekend, I spent a week in bed.

BRAHMACHARYA

Brahmacharya loosely translates as abstinence. Yes, it can be applied in the sexual sense, but it also means ridding your life of the things that drain you. As chronically-ill-forced-to-be-strong folk, we know that there are certain situations, activities, even people who deplete us. Our job is to recognize these things and abstain from engaging in certain activities or with certain individuals. To practice brahmicharya, I've had to abstain from many things. I have turned down writing jobs because I know they'd cause stress. I have avoided meeting friends for happy hours. I have walked away from unhealthy relationships. I continually reevaluate every situation in life to find where I need to walk away or abstain.

APARIGRAHA

Aparigraha translates as non-greed. This yama teaches us to let go, take only what we need, and keep only that which serves us in the moment. Aparigraha encourages us to let go of thoughts such as, *If I had X, I'd be happy.* Or, *If I wasn't sick, I'd have a better life.* What other thoughts and feelings can you let go? What are some things you can honestly say you don't need? As people living with chronic conditions, many of us need varying amounts of support, which is to be expected. At the same time, however, we don't want to rely too much on others. Aparigraha reminds us to recognize that the amount of energy others have to give us is also limited, and we can't be greedy and take it all. In that case, think of your specific needs and ask yourself: *When can I accept help from these saviors, but not drain their energy, too?* I have a very loving and supportive family, but I also recognize that they have their own lives to lead. While I may not be able to be there for them physically, I can be a listening ear or a shoulder to lean on. The road goes both ways and if I only take, then I become the greedy one.

NIYAMAS

After the yamas, come the niyamas, the ways to find discipline.

> Saucha – cleanliness
> Santosha – contentment
> Tapas – heat building
> Svadhyaya – self study
> Isvara pranidhana – surrendering

SAUCHA

Saucha means cleanliness. The simple way to look at this is keeping your house clean. But in our case, let's look at our house as our body. How can we nourish this body we inhabit to keep it clean? There may not be a cure for what ails us, but there are things we can practice that nurture and support our bodies. They will be different for each of us—it might be nutrition, physical therapy, talk therapy—but through this work we can discover what they are. For me, this means daily naps and cutting back on sugar. It means talking to my therapist and taking walks when I need movement in my life.

SANTOSHA

Santosha translates as contentment and being content with where you are. If there is one thing that living with lupus has taught me, it's that every day is different. I can't worry about tomorrow or fret over the things I couldn't do yesterday. Instead, santosha reminds me to be content with every single moment of the day. When you look at your life in moments, you can always find something to be content with. I encourage you to celebrate all the victories—from the small (I showered today!) to the big (I ran a half marathon!).

TAPAS

Tapas means to build heat. In a yoga class, this is literal heat to get your body warm and moving. In life, it's about working through the difficult moments to create change. The good thing is, living with illness has taught us a lot about working through the difficult times, and though it's not always easy or comfortable, we do know how to make it through. When I was lying on the floor screaming "Why me?" after my MS diagnosis, I didn't know how I'd continue to live. But I did and by working through the hard times—the nights of no sleep due to worry, the constant MRIs and other tests—I came out the other side stronger.

SVADHYAYA

Svadhyaya is self-study. It is about understanding your limits and constantly observing yourself. This is not to say that you constantly worry about new symptoms. Instead it's about learning what pain will help you grow, and what pains to avoid. It's a constant experiment of the body, observing how every action we take or don't take affects our well-being. Self-study is a perpetual loop of taking in feedback from your body and the world around you and learning from each experience. For me, it is about identifying the things that trigger my symptoms and the things that ease them. I've learned that if I don't get enough sleep my bone pain returns. I've learned that if I start to feel fatigued in the middle of a workout it's better to stop and walk away than to push through. I've learned that an Epsom salt bath is incredible for my joints as long as it's not too hot. Every day I learn something new by studying the effects my actions have on my body.

ISVARA PRANIDHANA

Isvara pranidhana is an acknowledgement that there is something out there bigger than us that guides and nurtures our whole self. Regardless of your belief system, isvara pranidhana is about understanding that we have no real control over anything. Though I've never been in AA, I always equate this niyama to the phrase, "Let go and let god." Even if you don't believe in god or a higher power, as someone living with illness, you constantly face the fact that you have no real control over anything. In order to move forward with our lives, we learn to let go of control and accept what is. We can certainly strive to feel better and be better, but there's also something to be said about the power of acceptance. Acceptance can free you from pain. For so long I fought to regain my old life. I fought for a body that could still compete in triathlons and swim miles in the ocean. But when I learned to accept that my body couldn't do all of this anymore, I discovered there were things I didn't know my body would enjoy—like Pilates and Hula-Hooping. Acceptance leads you away from the grief and pain that comes with fighting what is and allows you to discover something more fitting for who you are in the moment.

The yamas and the niyamas are some of the strongest guiding principles I use in my treatment plan, but that doesn't mean that's all there is to it. Beyond these two components of yoga, I also incorporate the other six limbs of ashtanga to complete the entire practice.

ASANA

Asana refers to the poses. It is everything from the complex, twist-yourself-into-a-pretzel poses to simply lying on your back with your eyes closed.

PRANAYAMA

Pranayama is the use of breath to calm the mind and connect to the body. There are entire practices devoted to different ways of breathing to produce a variety of results—from calmness, to heat, to learning to let go.

PRATYAHARA

Pratyahara is the process of turning inward. It's about creating an environment where there are no distractions—like turning off the lights so you can rest or turning off the internet so you can work.

DHARANA

Dharana is absolute focus. Pro athletes use dharana to win races and Super Bowls. In our case, we can use focus so that the pain can drift away. We can hone on the things that feel good or we can use a different sensation in our body to distract our minds from the pain. When my bone pain reaches an excruciating level, I turn to a TENS machine, which sends tiny electrical pulses to my muscles. It doesn't cure anything, but it serves as a point of focus that takes me away from dwelling on the pain and I feel it dissipate.

DHYANA

Dhyana is meditation, simply finding a singular point of focus. This can be your breath, movement, or a spot on the wall. The point is to find something to focus on so that your mind quiets and you can clear it. Meditation frees you from worry. Plus, science has proven that there's the added benefit of creating new neural pathways through meditation. That's great news for those of us with MS, brain injuries, or other illnesses that affect the brain.

SAMADHI

Samadhi is the perfect balance of all of these limbs. It is the ultimate now. It is enlightenment. A place where there is no worry about the future, no fret about the past. It is simply being here now. Samadhi is what we aim for with yoga. A place where we can appreciate the moment we are currently living in and be content in that space.

While you might be thinking, *How am I going to remember all these things?*—don't fret. They are easily incorporated into the practice as you'll see throughout the following chapters. With time you'll be able to apply the eight limbs of yoga to your life as if they were a natural extension of your being. The best part of yoga is that it is a practice. There is no mastery. There is no figuring it all out. There is no need to feel overwhelmed.

I'm here to teach you the small things you can do on a daily basis to bring these philosophies into practice. Which brings us to the first exercise.

A SIMPLE DAILY PRACTICE

A simple daily practice is just that. A simple list of things you can do daily no matter how you feel. These five things are breathe, move, close your eyes, meditate, and set an intention. They represent five of the limbs of ashtanga—pranayama, asana, pratyahara, dhyana, and dharana. You can do all five of them each day, or you can choose one or two or a few. The idea behind this is that you develop a habit to practice yoga every day.

BREATHE: Breath is pranayama. Whenever you need a little pick me up, or a reset, take a deep inhale through your nose, let your belly expand, hold for a second or two, then open your mouth and exhale. When I take the time to breathe, my demeanor changes. This change is different every time I do it, but nonetheless it is productive. By pausing and slowing down your inhale and your exhale, you are doing yoga.

MOVE: Movement is asana. Any amount of movement every day is great. One of my favorite trainers said it like this: "An object in motion, remains in motion." Movement is essential to our life force. If all you can do today is wiggle your toes, then do that. If you can walk, if you can do all the poses in this book, great. But you don't have to do anything big and impressive. The point is to move something and to do it daily.

CLOSE YOUR EYES: Closing your eyes helps you learn to shut out the outside world and focus inwards, what yogis call pratyahara. To start, close your eyes and imagine staring at a blank chalkboard. Don't write anything on it, don't try to move it, just let it sit there empty. When you picture an empty board, it makes it hard for you to worry or judge or leap into the what-ifs of the future or fret about the past. The point of closing your eyes and focusing on a blank board is to focus on nothing. When you focus on nothing you free yourself from wondering what the outside world thinks of you.

MEDITATE: Meditation, i.e., dhyana, is simply drawing your attention to one single point of focus. Closing your eyes and focusing inwards (pratyahara) is the prep for meditation. It clears space and allows you to shut out the outside world so you can draw your attention to one point of focus. That's meditation. It's not an impossible task. Simply pick something you can focus on—real or imagined—and see how long you can keep your attention drawn to it. There are no set limits that say you have to meditate for minutes or hours. Focus as long as you can focus. If that's ten seconds, so be it. With time you'll be able to last for longer periods.

SET AN INTENTION: To help us face the unpredictability of our lives, every day we can set an intention for ourselves. At the beginning of each day, think about what you need to thrive over the next 24 hours, then make that your intention. Perhaps your intention reinforces how you feel or perhaps it's an intention to help you get out of a funk. Maybe your intention is, "Today I will be kind to my body," or maybe you're feeling run down and you say, "My body is a powerhouse." It doesn't matter what you say, find something that makes sense to you. When you set an intention, you create a purpose for that day and that gives you motivation to keep moving forward. It gives you absolute focus, or dharana.

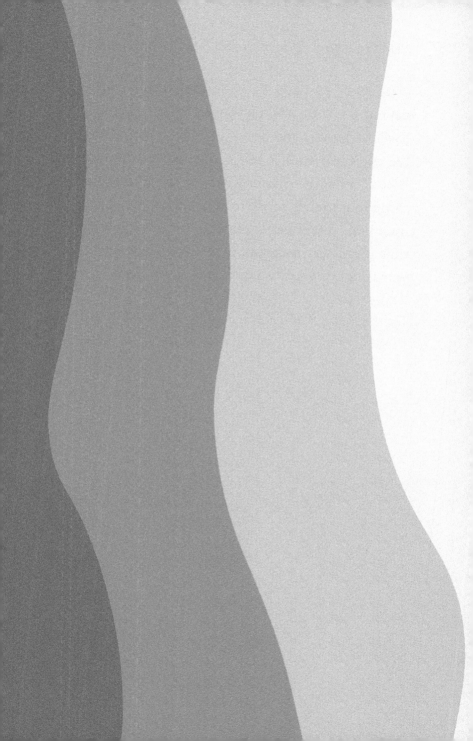

CHAPTER THREE

Be Here Now

If you grew up in the '70s, you might know the phrase from the eponymous book by Ram Dass: *Be Here Now*. However, if you're slightly younger than that, or came of age during the Instagram era, you might have seen it on a shirt, as a meme, or heard it in a yoga class or the Ray LaMontagne song. Regardless, the phrase is a good reminder of what this yoga practice is all about and the perfect place to begin your own practice.

The first yoga sutra says, *Yoga is now.* If you understand that and can apply it to your life on a consistent basis—and by consistent I mean every waking second—then that's all there is to it! No need to study further. No need to pass Go. However, if you're like 99.999999 percent of the population, you'll need a little bit of help.

The good thing is, I believe we all have an advantage here. When you live in pain or constantly have to track your symptoms, you are forced to live in the moment. Chronic illness pushes you to pay attention to what is happening every second of the day. I don't know about you, but it's a rare moment where my diseases are not a thought in my head. Whether those thoughts are good or bad, they are a constant.

In some ways I believe pain is a gift to put us in that *be here now* state. I'm not saying I like living in pain, but I do like looking at the bright side of things. I like the challenge of taking the terrible things I go through and figuring out a way to spin them positively. Next time you're in pain, why not try looking at it as an exercise in living in the moment. This is not easy by any means, but it's something I try to work towards. I think of the pain as a reminder that if I stay in the present moment, I don't have to worry about what will happen tomorrow (will I wake up and be unable to walk?), or next year (will I enter a flare?), or five years down the road (will I experience kidney failure?). I don't have to lament the things I used to do, like swimming miles in the hot sun. If I focus on the pain, which can range from mildly annoying to tear inducing, I don't have the mental capacity to think about anything but the present moment. I can then embrace the moment as a gift.

Now, before you think I'm up on my soapbox preaching something that seems impossible, let me be clear: Try as I might, living in the now is freaking hard.

I always think I'm in the now. I always believe I have it figured out, that I'm absolutely zen and I don't need to do any more work—but then here's what happens. On good days, when my body feels amazing, I get excited. I get pumped up thinking, *This is it!* The drugs are lessening my symptoms, the diet changes are actually working, the sleep is helping, and I'm finally on the upswing. I settle into that moment and enjoy how great it feels. Then seconds later I find myself fantasizing about the next day, and the next. I fantasize about how I'm going to go for a long swim or walk two miles on the beach... *How I'm going to be able to do the yoga poses I used to do... How I can return to my regular routine and feel excited about each day.* The thoughts go on and on and though it's great to imagine that future, that future is no longer my present and I'm suddenly out of the moment. While there's no real danger in that—we all need something to look forward to—the problem arises when tomorrow arrives and the future I envisioned is nothing like the present I'm experiencing. If, after a good day, where I've fantasized about the great future ahead, I can't concentrate to write another word or I have to leave a workout early or chewing becomes an exhausting task, I find myself looking back at the past and I will beat myself up over it. Why didn't I just savor the moment? Why didn't I enjoy the fact that yesterday I was free of pain—so much so that I showered, dressed, and even put on makeup? When I get into this line of questioning, I look at yesterday as a failure. *I ruined a good day*, I tell myself. Then I go on a shame spiral because I feel like I've let myself down. I'm mad at what I did the day before, and when I look at the future, all I can see is a poor outlook. *I can't live like this forever*, I say, *I'm never going to get better.* Then I curse yesterday. I shouldn't have eaten that piece of cake. I should've only walked one mile instead of two. I shouldn't have done so many things. I do all this bargaining in my head between the past and the present, trying to figure out how to fix the moment. But the moment can't be fixed when this negative feedback loop plays on repeat.

However, if I can come back to Patanjali's yoga and remember that *yoga is now*. I can bring myself out of the bad loop. It's never easy, but to come back to the moment, I turn to my bag of yoga tricks—those trusty eight limbs of yoga.

Sometimes escaping that negativity is as simple as taking a deep breath (pranayama) through my nose, filling up my lungs with air and letting my belly expand, then opening my mouth and sighing it out. Sometimes I need to close my eyes and focus on the concept of ahimsa—do no harm—and remind myself not to beat myself up over my current state. But sometimes I need to do a little more. Sometimes I have to get a little physical.

Though movement, or asana, is just one limb on the eight limbs of yoga, it is still essential. Because movement is something we all have experience with, the poses throughout the book are meant to be a place to start to help you achieve the purpose of each chapter. You can look at the poses as a quick way to help you reach each state until the philosophies become innate to your everyday life. To reach that state of *be here now* you can use our first yoga asana or pose—savasana.

SAVASANA

Even if you've never done yoga, you've probably heard of savasana. It's that great pose that ends every class where you lie on your back and close your eyes. What people don't know is that it's a great pose to do any time. You don't have to have completed 60 minutes of a strong flow to enjoy this pose. In fact, I urge you to use this pose not only as a way to bring yourself into the present moment when you're stuck in that negative feedback loop, but also as a way to start and end your day. The great part is, most of us already start and end our days in bed or at least lying down in some manner, so you probably have a lot of experience here. See? Look at that: You're already a yogi.

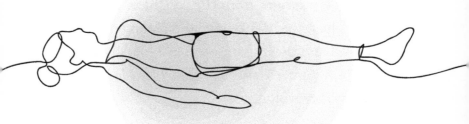

INSTRUCTIONS

While it might seem that a pose where you're simply lying on your back with your eyes closed needs no further explanation, there's a little more to savasana.

Here's what I want you to do. Find a place where you can lie comfortably on your back. If you're in pain of any form, do whatever you need to do to feel as comfortable as possible. If this means sitting up or lying on your side, then by all means do that. The point of this pose is to eliminate as many distractions as possible so that you can tune into your body. I like to lie with my arms alongside me palms face up, but sometimes when I'm feeling incredibly scattered and my monkey mind is running, I'll place one hand over my heart and the other on my belly. There's something about the gentle pressure from the weight of my hand on my chest that's calming, and feeling my belly move up and down with each breath is reassuring. It's a gentle reminder that I am still here. Alive and breathing.

Once you're comfortable (in whatever relaxed state works for you), close your eyes and breathe normally. With each breath, begin to pay attention to what's happening in your body. Is there tightness or tension anywhere? Are you in pain? Is it difficult to breathe? Is your heart racing? Are your legs achy or twitchy? Whatever is going on, simply observe. Do not judge any part of this. Simply say, *Yes, my legs hurt.* Or, *My neck feels tight.* Don't try to decipher what's causing what, or lament what you did wrong yesterday, or try to determine if your meds are working, or decide that you shouldn't have had that glass of wine. The point is to acknowledge the current state of your body. Whatever that is, is fine.

This will most likely be difficult to do at first, especially if you're used to jumping to the past or the future, but I promise it will get easier. The more you do it, the longer you'll be able to lie there and observe without placing judgment on any part of the body. It will simply be an acknowledgment of where you're at in that particular moment. Later, you can use your observations to help you move through the day, but in these five minutes when you're lying here, simply be. There is no rush to get up and go. This is your time to check in with yourself and **be here now.**

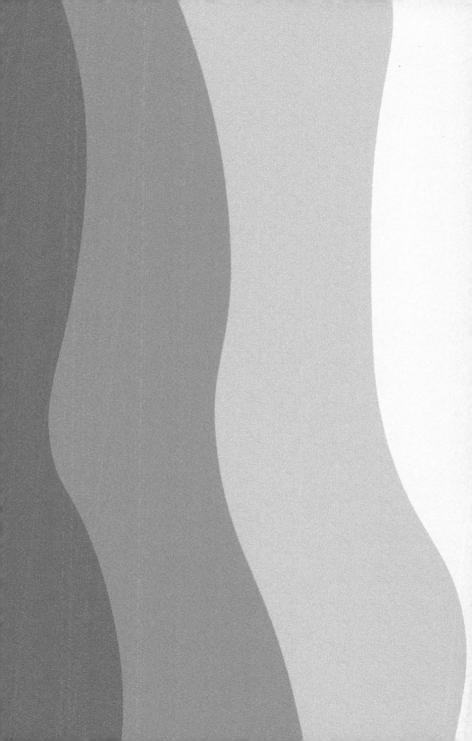

CHAPTER FOUR

Give Props to Yourself

Living with illness of any kind is difficult. We struggle. We cry. We get mad: Mad at our bodies. Mad at the world. Mad at god and the universe for giving us these diseases. Sometimes the anger gets so bad that we take it out on ourselves. We beat ourselves up and blame ourselves for everything we're going through. We spew hatred at our bodies as if they're the worst employee in the world and we believe they're never going to listen unless we shout at them. So, we scream and shout but then they ignore us or act out and do even worse things. They give us pain, and fatigue, and difficulty concentrating and working. In these moments, when my body refuses to listen and everything seems hopeless, I don't want to have to deal with the flesh I've been given anymore. My bone-crushing fatigue gets so bad sometimes that I can't imagine walking through another day. Living in pain makes me break down in tears quite often, and I struggle to see my way out of it. It's too much work. It's too much effort. It's draining. It's saddening. When I get caught in these moments, they can last for days or weeks, even months. Yet, every time I reach these points of despair, I remind myself that there is a way through. I find my footing and push to find something that can support me. This is when I give myself props. In the asana practice of yoga, props are physical objects to make poses more accessible. In life, props are the pep talks to keep us going. In life with chronic illness, we need both. We may need mobility aids or other objects to move us through our daily lives, and we need to cheer ourselves on.

Propping ourselves up with words may sound like an abstract idea that's too self-congratulatory,

but it doesn't need to be. Often, when we can
sit and listen to our body, we will be told exactly
what we need.

One day, after a particularly difficult time—hello,
not being able to walk upstairs without needing a
two-hour nap—I decided I'd had enough berating
myself. I wanted to give my body a break. I was
tired of fighting. I realized that my body was not a
bad employee that I wanted to fire, put down, or
embarrass. It was my business partner, and if we
were going to succeed, we had to work together
harmoniously and support one another. We are
partners who must have each other's back. We
can have our off days, our spats—but at the end of
the day, we are in this together.

As I lay in bed that night with those thoughts in
my head, I instinctively placed my hand in the
middle of my chest and suddenly out of nowhere
I said, *I love and respect you.* I hadn't planned on
setting any sort of intention or talking to myself,
it simply felt right in the moment. When those
words left my mouth, I immediately felt a sense
of calm. My body relaxed. The tenseness I carried

in my shoulders dissipated. I hadn't learned to say this to myself from any teacher or book I'd read, it was simply something that came to me in that moment, yet it was exactly what I needed. In essence, it was pratyahara, a turning inward to reflect on the fact that beating myself up, not practicing ahimsa, was doing me harm, and it led me to say those words. *I love and respect you.* Working through the difficult moments of hating my body and the turmoil it was putting me through had taught me a lesson. I learned to step back and allow my body to do what it needs to do. Every night since that moment, I've said those five words. And guess what? My body has responded to my encouragement. I have less days of pain. I experience less fatigue. I'm happier. Sure, I still have moments of upset, but now I know I can get out of them. In these situations, words are my props.

If you'd told 16-year-old me that I'd have to deal with MS and lupus and all the symptoms, tests, and fears that come along with the diseases, I would've questioned how I could ever make it through. Then, I wouldn't have had an answer.

But today, I do. The answer is one step at a time, one breath at a time, one small mantra of five words at a time—*I love and respect you.* These are my props in life in dealing with disease.

Sometimes I have to place my hand over my heart and remind myself of everything I've been through—the countless MRIs, days of endless fatigue, the tears I've cried into the shoulder of my dad, deep bone pain. I have to give myself props for all that. In the dark moments, I place my hand on my heart center and speak kindly. Words, breath, movement—all help me to move through this difficult life in a mindful manner.

The props in yoga are meant to do the same. In a yoga studio, physical props aid students in finding their footing. Props are objects that help students move into poses. These can be blocks, bolsters, straps, even blankets or chairs. They're meant to help you move through in the smartest, most-aware way.

Over the years of teaching, I've watched many people struggle through class. I offer props to help them with a pose—like a block to bring the ground closer to their hand—but they refuse. They think they aren't doing the pose right, and that using a prop means they are taking the easy way out. In reality, choosing to use props is precisely the opposite. When you use a prop, you are fully aware of your situation and know exactly what you need in that moment.

Learning what you need in any given moment is one of the biggest elements you can take away from a yoga practice. Choosing props, whether they be words or physical objects, demonstrates that you fully understand the situation at hand. In class, students often look at props as a weakness or an inability to fully do the pose. They see them as an unnecessary helping hand, but props are not training wheels. In fact, they're an intelligent decision. The student who chooses the prop is the person who knows their body and listens to it. When we listen and honor what our body asks for, we make it through the rough times.

As people dealing with chronic illness, we've been forced to listen to our body because it constantly screams at us. *Don't do that. Stop. You aren't going to feel good later.* And while we might try to ignore these signs, we eventually reach a point where we have to listen. With chronic illness, we have to be fully aware. We have to choose the mobility aid that lessens our fatigue, or the brace that helps with pain. In yoga, the most advanced practitioner is the one who listens to this voice. The beauty is, you already know this voice.

As you begin your yoga practice, you may need to use props—and that's okay. There is no need to buy any fancy equipment. You're more than welcome to do so, but it's not necessary. You can make do with what you have in your house. Props are any objects that can support you in your movement. They can be pillows, a wall or other supporting structure, towels, or a rope. Props can be your bed or a couch or a chair. The props you find are anything that will ease you into a space of awareness.

FORWARD FOLD (UTTANASANA)

The forward fold is a gentle way to wake up the backs of your legs. You can do this seated or lying on your back with props.

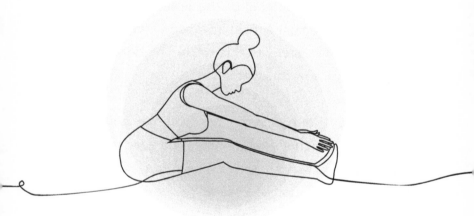

INSTRUCTIONS

To do the forward fold seated, sit up tall on the floor in an L-shape. Legs straight in front of you. Flex your feet, place your hands next to your hips with arms straight. If this already feels like an enormous stretch in your hamstrings, stop there.

If you need more, walk your hands forward until you feel a slight stretch at the back of your legs.

To do this on your back, grab a towel or a long sleeve shirt or a rope and hook it around the soles of your feet as you extend them towards the sky. To ease the stretch, lower your legs towards the ground. The point isn't that you're in a perfect L-shape, but that you can keep your legs straight and the rest of your body relaxed.

You can also do this pose by using a wall as your prop. Lie down on your back and place your legs up the wall to come into an L-shape. If it's too much of a stretch, you can always bend your knees a bit or back away from the wall.

Whatever version you choose, **give yourself props**, for showing up and beginning this journey.

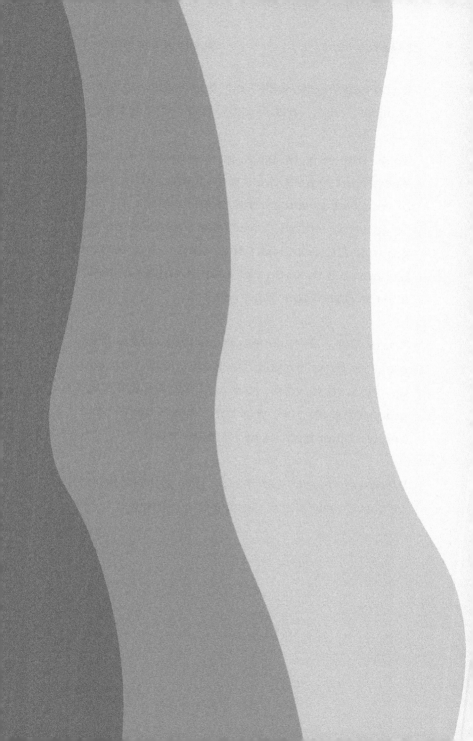

CHAPTER **FIVE**

Slow Down and Embrace the Beginner Within

I often hear from people—friends, family, coworkers—who've never tried yoga that they are scared. They fear they are not flexible enough, or are afraid that others will stare at them because they don't know what they're doing, or they're terrified that they'll be laughed at. My job as a teacher is to tell them that no one's noticing, and no one cares. Yoga isn't about being perfect or knowing everything, it's about trusting that you will eventually get there. Where that "there" is for you, that is part of the journey. Whether that means you can touch your toes one day, balance on your hands, or simply learn how to breathe through the difficult times, your "there" is unique to you and only you. The same is true living with illness.

I've been through difficult diagnoses twice now and I'm here to tell you that I'm still looking for my "there." A doctor doesn't just say one day, "You have lupus, take this drug," and the next day you're fine. There's a process. Sometimes that process takes a year, sometimes it's ten years, sometimes it's for life. Part of that ongoing process is the science of the drugs and the treatment plan, and part of it is the grief process.

There's a tendency when we're first diagnosed to want answers. We want them right now. Immediately. We want relief. We want a cure. We want to be in our new normal. We want to rush through all the difficult parts and get back to the living part. But, here's the problem: If we really want to reach a point of contentment (santosha) with our new normal, we have to move through the difficult first. We don't get to rush through life to reach the now that is easy and comfortable. We have to move through all the steps of grief first.

We have to allow ourselves to work through the grief—to be in denial, to get angry, to bargain with ourselves or a higher power, and to be sad and depressed—before we can reach a place of acceptance. We have to be okay with the fact that acceptance may be temporary and ever changing and that we're going to constantly be moving through these stages. We have to acknowledge that things will never move at the pace we want them to. This is tapas in its purest form, moving through the difficult to find the things that make us stronger and more resilient.

When I was first told I had MS, I wanted to go out and do something grand. I had it in my head that I would write a book about my experiences. I believed it would take me six months to complete. Then, it'd be published and I'd help people the world over. My book would be my mark on the world. I thought that since I had a plan that focused on the positives of my diagnosis that I could bypass all the uncomfortable stages of mourning the loss of my "healthy" self. But this was not my reality. I started writing my book, yes, but I also spent hours on end sleeping on my couch or Googling possible symptoms and worrying about my future. I cried to no one late at night in my apartment. I bargained that if I changed my diet (hello, organic!) and worked out every day, that the powers that be would leave me in control of what happens to my body. I believed that I had tricked the system. That because I was writing a book that would help people live with their disease at a young age, that meant I didn't have to deal with my reality. The same reality landed me in the ER after a botched spinal tap, and made the guy I decided not to date anymore text me horrible messages saying he was glad I broke up with him so that now he could find a woman who would actually live to see her kids grow up. I thought I could escape my difficult reality by doing good in the world. I truly believed I could negotiate my way out of the horrible feelings I had around my diagnosis. I believed that if I kept plowing through, spinning everything into a positive, that I would reach a "normal" state again. I believed I could barter my way into power. I was dead wrong.

Looking back, I can see that I had to go through all the phases of grief in order to come out all right. I had to live through each difficult moment in order to write a book about my experiences. That book, *Love Sick*, took eight years to complete. It would be another two years after publication before it started to leave a mark on the world. But that mark is finally starting to become permanent and while that's wonderful, I'm also over here dealing with my second devastating diagnosis. With lupus, I'm having to live through these stages of grief all over again. And again, I feel this strong urge to rush through the difficult, even though I know deep down that I can't, that it is all part of the process of becoming who I am meant to be. But that doesn't mean I'm not going to try—futile or not—because that is also who I am.

When I picked up yoga for the pure physicality of it, I was determined to be good right away. As a former athlete, I was used to being able to begin any physical activity and be decent at it. Even though I struggled in my first class, I didn't want to do all the work that the teachers kept talking about. I wanted to show up to class day after day and become better. But I soon realized that if I wanted to balance on my hands in crow pose or nail a handstand, I would have to move through other poses first. There is a method to every part of this practice and each asana or pose is built on another. You have to start from the bottom to create the strength to hold those fancy poses I kept seeing my teachers rock. I didn't know it at the time, but yoga was teaching me to move slowly and enjoy the process.

With yoga the emphasis is on slowing down and observing, not the rush to achievement. There's no need to reach the "advanced" poses right away. The same is true with our selves. There's no need to become the face of your disease or go out and do something grand. If your goal is to touch your toes or balance in tree pose, or feel normal, or tell a friend what you're going through, or write a book, or start an online course to help others deal with their disease, you have to do all the work to get there.

When I first started practicing yoga, one of my teachers constantly said, "Enjoy this time, you're only a beginner once." I never appreciated the phrase. *Who cares?* I thought. *I want to be big and impressive. I want to be an advanced yogi, this beginner phase isn't going to last long. Why waste my time being a beginner? That's for losers.* I was determined to push right through. I wanted everything here and now. What I now see and understand is that the beginning phase is just as important as the continuation phase. It's a time and place to learn, to reflect on who you are.

Who I am now and who I was before my diagnoses are fundamentally the same, and yet they are eons apart. Embracing your beginner phase is like embracing all the firsts of your life without fear. Firsts can be exciting, but they can also be incredibly scary, full of the unknown. The first time our doctor utters the words that form our diagnosis we are thrown for a loop. We are terrified and absolutely worried for our futures. Unfortunately, this worry doesn't always go away. In fact, I am still scared nearly every morning. Sometimes that fear lasts all day, sometimes it's fleeting. But there is always a moment of fear when I first wake up and check in with my body—is today a good day or a bad day? Will the day be easy or hard? I never know until I open my eyes. Living with an autoimmune disease means that I cannot predict my day to day; the only thing I can control is how I react to it all. And let me be clear, my reactions are not always pretty.

Sometimes they are knee jerk, f-this kind of reactions and other times they're defeatist, like this is what I've been given and there's no way I'll ever feel better. In these times, I have to remember the yama, asteya—not to steal. I have to remember that I don't need to covet all the things it appears everyone else around me gets to do or experience that I can't. I have to remember that I am moving through life at my own pace now and to compare myself to others is a futile attempt at making things better. Even so, this is a practice easier said than done.

To help me get out of this place of wanting to be healthy like others, I have learned to sit and reflect and move as needed. A great place to reflect on your reactions to the daily, weekly, monthly, and yearly changes in your body is in easy pose.

EASY POSE (SUKHASANA)

I'm not sure why this translates as easy pose, because for so many of us this is not an easy pose. The classic instruction is to sit cross-legged like you did in kindergarten. However, many of our bone structures don't allow this, especially if we're a tad bit older than five.

For the purposes of this book, I will instruct the classic pose but also give plenty of options to make adjustments so you can be comfortable and sit with ease.

The point of easy pose is to find a place where you can sit comfortably and be alert. You want to

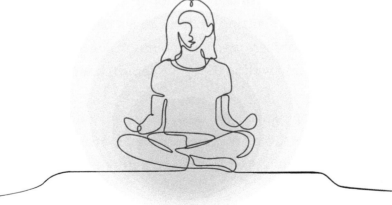

engage enough of your body so that you actively have to sit up tall, but not so much that you are exhausting yourself.

INSTRUCTIONS

Find a place where you can sit without a lot of distractions. You don't want your attention to be diverted to your dog, your spouse, a buzzing phone. Once you find a quiet place, sit up tall on your sitz bones and cross your shins in front of you. Cross your shins in the middle so that you're not pulling them into your body and instead are letting them relax.

If your knees are really high off the ground, grab a couple of pillows and stack them underneath your knees until they're supported and it feels easy to sit. If sitting up tall causes pain in your back or forces you to use too much energy, then sit against a wall so that your spine is supported.

If having your legs crossed is so incredibly uncomfortable and you can't even fathom how anyone could do this, then straighten your legs in front of you in a way that makes sense. This might mean that they're perfectly straight and perpendicular to your hips, or it might mean that you bend your knees and put your feet on the ground and sit against the wall. Remember, this pose is called easy pose, not because it's easy in its formation but because it calls on you to find the position that is easy for your body in this moment. Don't be surprised if this changes from day to day.

After you find your easy pose, close your eyes and take five deep breaths. As you're breathing, think of one word you can focus on for the day and with every inhale say that word to yourself.

For example, on the days where I feel drained and fatigued but need to finish an assignment and have to muster a little energy, I might come back to my trusty "powerhouse." That word makes me feel powerful and it serves as a reminder that I am strong. It reminds me that despite how my body might feel in that moment, it has persevered through so much and it truly is a powerhouse. And then there are days when I need to honor and respect my limitations and my word might be "peace" or "rest," as a reminder that it's okay to not keep pushing through. There is no right or wrong word to say. All of this is personal to you, so choose a word that makes sense in your now.

After you take your five breaths (and if you're enjoying them please take more), I want you to add a little movement to your body by twisting. Sit up tall, take your right hand behind you and place it on the ground, a pillow, or some other prop if the ground feels far away. Cross your left hand over your body and place it to the outside of the right side of your body and twist your spine from there.

Pay attention to how you feel—keep it easy and comfortable, don't rush anything. Ideally, you should stay in this twist for at least five breaths. Then repeat on the other side. However, I have to be honest, some days this is doable and other days this feels too constricting on my lungs (hi, MS hug). If this is the case, you can do these twists gently: Maybe all you do is turn your body slightly, and do them one breath per movement. Where ever you are, settle into the moment, **slow down,** and **embrace the beginner within.**

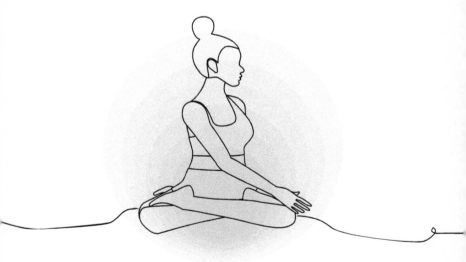

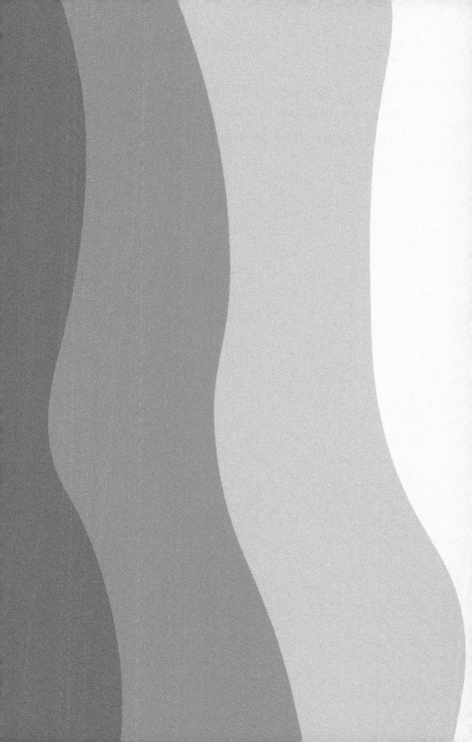

CHAPTER SIX

Practice Makes Life

In yoga, you never reach a state of perfection because yoga was never meant to be something mastered. Instead, yoga was created as a *practice*, a daily discipline to help us deal with the constant inevitable changes of life. Life is not linear and change is the one thing we can all count on being consistent. The world around us changes. The environment changes. Our friendships, our careers, and our entire beings are constantly changing. This would be true whether or not we are dealing with chronic illness. We age, become stressed by life events, gain strength, and lose strength. We will be happy and sad, up and down.

Many of us will never be cured of our illnesses. Even if we are, we'll still be faced with the fact that we could get any number of diseases. I thought I had my health under control with MS, then I was hit with lupus. And the truth is, there will probably be something else I'll face in the future, and that's simply a part of living. My health is a practice, ever changing, which means I am ever adjusting. Through yoga I have learned to take things day by day. I have had to embrace the unknown and see it as an opportunity. Every time I'm faced with another blow to my health, I view it as a chance to learn something new about myself, my body, and my coping methods.

With lupus I've learned to become hyperaware of certain signals my body sends. These signals originally felt like constant symptoms and, in fact, they were. But as I learned to adjust to life with lupus, I came to discover that my deep bone pain was not just a symptom, but also a sign that I was overdoing it. Before I was diagnosed and began treatment, that bone pain was constant in my legs and arms. After I began taking the drugs my doctor prescribed, that pain began to become less constant. Over the course of a year, the pain subsided greatly, but it still appears. And now I recognize it as a reminder to slow down.

When that pain comes on, I now pause to take inventory of everything happening in my life at that moment. Have I been pushing myself too hard at the gym? Not getting enough sleep? Did I miss a dose of my drug? I run through the litany of possible causes and try to narrow it down to one, but I also stay open to the fact that it could be something completely new causing the pain this time. I do my best to check in and figure out what is causing the pain so that I can take steps to alleviate it.

The point here isn't that I'm a perfect scientist who has the correct answers every time, but that I'm paying attention and training myself to become more aware of what's happening around me that affects my health. Being aware of our bodies can mean regular doctor appointments, frequent testing, and other science-backed tracking. But checking in can also mean looking at the subtle changes that happen within the confines of our bodies and limitations of our disease.

Two years into my lupus diagnosis, I now know that one of the biggest factors in the state of my health is the sun—but it took me awhile to figure this out. Even though my rheumatologist had told me to avoid prolonged periods in the sun, I didn't think it was that big of a deal. Sure, I thought, some lupus patients have problems with the sun, but I've been playing outdoors since I was a little girl. No way could the sun be causing any of my pain and fatigue. But the more time I spent in the sun, the worse I felt. I broke out in rashes when I played a four-hour round of golf in the middle of the day. I had to nap for five hours after swimming in the sun for one hour. I got dizzy when I sat on my porch for twenty minutes in the middle of the day. My fatigue worsened over time despite the meds that were supposed to help. I worried about not getting any better after the initial start of my medication, but it turned out the sun was the culprit. It took me a year and a half to become serious about avoiding the sun; but now that I have, I feel 90 percent better. For the first year post diagnosis, I tried everything from diet to exercise to make myself feel better when all I had to do was pay attention to how I felt when I spent long periods in the sun. The sun was at the root of many of my problems.

At my last rheumatology appointment, my doctor had a resident with him who he was training. "Are you avoiding the sun?" my doctor asked. "Definitely!" I responded. Then he went on to explain to the resident that lupus patients will often enter a flare or have symptoms of a flare for three weeks after sun exposure. I had never heard this, nor read it on any of the lupus sites online, but I knew it was true from my own experiences—and I kind of wished he'd been more stern when he'd cautioned me originally. But I suppose that this was part of my practice too, to learn on my own.

In my early days of practicing yoga, when I was obsessed with mastering the poses, I was very aware of the differences in my practice from day to day. Because I didn't understand that there was no "mastering" of the poses, I was determined to figure it out. *Why was my balance off today? Did I not get enough sleep? Did I run too far the day before? Was I too worried about the work I had to return to after class?* I didn't know it at the time, but what

I was really training myself to do was to be aware.

This awareness later translated to my life with chronic illness. As my practice progressed, and I learned that it was more about the practice than anything else, I started to care less about the mastery and used every moment on my mat as a teaching experience.

The same is now true with my health. When I take the time to observe and reflect on how I feel, I learn something new about my disease and how it affects my body. To help us deal with the changes of living with illness, we can rely on yoga's teachings that we take the time to constantly check in our selves. What is our physical state in the moment? Our mental state? What are the things we can do to embrace the current state or work to improve the future state? How can we be more aware of who we are in any given moment?

Doctors are incredible beings and when you find the right one who you trust deeply, they can be incredibly beneficial to your health. But even the greatest doctor in the world won't know exactly how it feels to live in your body every minute of the day. Only you can.

Knowing your body intimately is the point of the practice, but also the benefit to living with chronic illness. One of the poses, or set of poses I should say, that I really like to help me check in on the state of my body is cat/cow.

CAT/COW (MARJARYASANA/BITLASANA)

The cat/cow set of poses is a big movement of the spine. In that movement, you can feel every bit of your body—where things ache, where they feel good. You can even use these poses to check in on your heart and lungs, the tightness of your muscles, the mobility of your joints.

In a traditional yoga class, you will often find cat/cow towards the beginning of class as a way to "wake up" the spine.

INSTRUCTIONS

Come to your hands and knees. This can be done on your bed, on the carpet, or on a yoga mat. If you're on the ground and your knees feel like they're digging into the floor, place a light pillow or a blanket underneath them as padding.

Spread your fingers wide and press evenly through all ten digits and the palms of your hands. Keep your hands active and engaged. On an inhale, drop your belly to the floor as you let your hips rise. Begin to look up but don't strain your neck. It should feel like you're rolling your shoulders back to open your chest.

As you exhale, press firmly into your hands and draw your belly button into your spine. Allow your gaze to come down between your hands as you relax your neck. Keep pressing into your hands and rounding your back so that you create space between your shoulder blades.

Keep repeating this movement with your breath: Inhale and drop your belly as you look up; exhale, press into your hands, and round your spine as you look down.

As you move through these two poses, pay attention to where things feel tight or awkward or painful. Don't press through the pain but simply note it as a reminder of where you are today. Remember, we're only using these poses to gain insight into our bodies. Nothing has to be perfect. It is simply a practice, and **practice is life**.

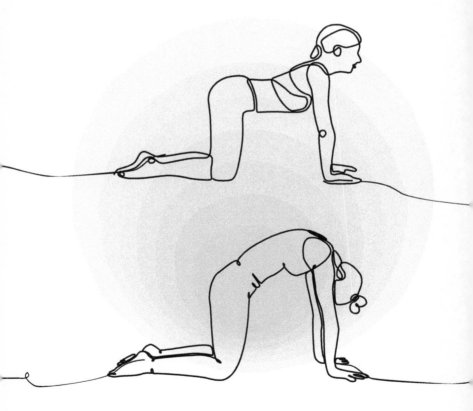

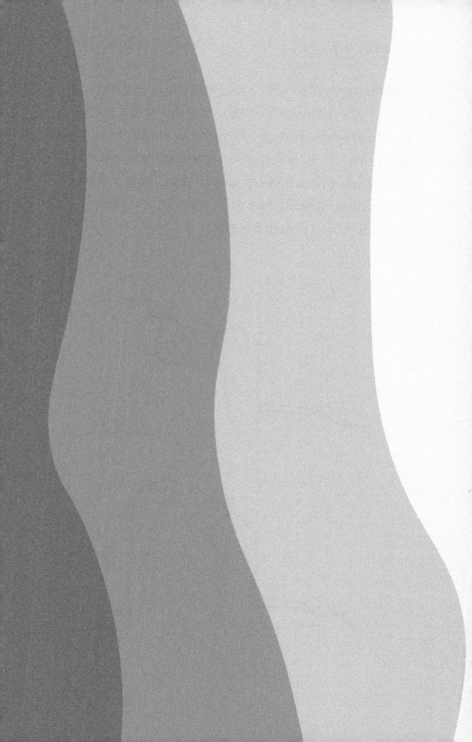

CHAPTER **SEVEN**

Listen to Your Body

O ften, the concept of listening to your body sounds too woo-woo, like in order to listen to your body you have to have some sort of psychic powers. But the truth is, it's really simple. We were born to understand our body's needs. At birth we innately knew how to listen to what we needed and literally cry out for it. We cried when we were hungry. We cried when we needed our diaper changed. We cried when we wanted to be held. Our bodies knew exactly what they needed and how to get it.

Even today, the body still sends real signals to the brain to tell it what it needs. These signals can be completely overt, like a growling stomach when we're hungry, or more subtle, like a drop in energy signaling that we need to rest. The problem with these subtle signals is that we've become so conditioned to ignore them by society that it's hard to hear them. Rest is not usually looked at as something crucial to our success. The person who works an 80-hour week is always praised and glorified over the one who leaves a few hours early on a Tuesday because they can feel fatigue setting in and they understand that they've maxed out their brain and any work they do from that point forward will need to be redone the next day so might as well leave now while they're ahead and face the task the following day when they're recharged. No, society says that the person who learns to ignore and overcome their body's signals is the one who becomes successful.

If you were an athlete growing up or even in your later years, you probably learned to live by the no pain, no gain attitude. The sentiment was clear: If you didn't push past your limits, there was no way you'd get better.

At my first "grown up" job, the idea that I had to push my limits to be recognized as good was very apparent. One day, I came to work deathly ill, loaded up on DayQuil and struggling to get by. I did this for four days straight. Calling in sick was never an option. Luckily, my boss allowed me to go home early during that time and let me leave at 7 p.m. each day. When the weekend arrived, I ended up in urgent care with severe bronchitis. I missed my sister's 21st birthday. I missed spending time with my family. But I thought nothing of it, because who was I to listen to my body? That was not the important voice here. My boss, my career, my paycheck—all took precedent over anything my body had to say. It makes me sad to think about it now, but during that time, pushing through was life.

In fact, I took the concept of no pain, no gain, no rest for the weary with me straight to working my way up as a writer and later into my yoga training. As part of my training to become a teacher, I had to create a daily practice. Five days a week for an hour and a half each day, I would put my body through a sequence of poses I'd created. I pushed myself to the limit every single day. Did I get better? Sure. I was awesome at balancing on my hands in crazy contorted positions. But was I listening to my body? Absolutely not. My back was in constant pain. I had no energy. I felt like crap. But I kept pushing forward because I had been so conditioned to listen not to my body but to what the outside world was telling me to do. *No pain, no gain!* it shouted, and I heard it.

All of this pushing took place after I was told I had MS but before I'd ever had to work through the debilitating symptoms of lupus. This was also before I truly immersed myself in the practice of yoga and began to understand the true breadth of the practice.

I now see my lupus diagnosis as a wake-up call to learn to listen to my body again. Despite what we've all been conditioned to do, the good news is that living with chronic illness has already begun to waken the part of you that knows how to listen to your body. While I may have been living in the fog of pushing my body to its limits, I could still hear enough to say "something's not right" and tell my doctor my symptoms. My guess is it is your knowledge of your body that helped you find a diagnosis and the right doctor in the first place.

I hear horror stories of those who knew something was wrong with their health but were brushed off and told all their symptoms were in their head. When the medical establishment says things like that to us, it makes us doubt our ability to listen to our body. But I'm here to tell you that you are already an expert in listening to your body. Now you get to channel that expertise into something that will make you feel better. You might currently be in a state where all you hear are subtle whispers saying something's wrong, but with time and practice you can reach a state where you will hear your body's cries for help, assistance, love, and caring loud and clear.

By looking inward, practicing pratyahara, you can slow down and observe the subtle signals your body sends. You can ask it questions. *Do you need rest? Nourishment? Love? Patience? Understanding?* These can be said to yourself or even out loud. When you can put yourself into a safe place—where you're working towards being in the now, and don't have to worry about a deadline or a boss thinking you're weak for not powering through your illness—you can simply observe. Then you can use svadhyaya, the practice of self-study, and experiment on your own body and its needs. When I first experienced that excruciating leg pain, I thought it was because I'd eaten too much gluten. I turned to Dr. Google and decided that my brain knew best. But the truth was my body knew best. And when I experimented by eliminating gluten and found no correlation and the pain didn't subside, I knew it was time to look at another factor. I tried doing more stretches, but that didn't work either. Finally, I tried backing off of my daily routine and slowing down and resting more. It was then that I finally felt a sense of relief. Sure, the disease-modifying drug I was on was helping, but the bigger factor was that I was learning to build in more rest into my day. When I finally found this answer, I began to feel relief. For now, this is my solution to the bone pain in my legs. This may no longer work one day, and I may have to conduct more experiments to find out what will. Until then, I will keep listening and evolving.

Just as my yoga practice today looks far different than it did when I was 28, 29, and even 30, my body's signals will continuously change and ask for different things. A baby grows up and stops crying when they're hungry. Instead, they learn to ask, "What's for dinner?" This is the same process for you. You will learn to go from primal instincts to taking feedback and forming intelligent hypotheses in order to ask for what you need. Your needs will always vary, but the process of listening to your body and tuning into what it needs will always require the same amount of introspection, experimentation, and contemplation.

Today, the answer to your pain may be that you need to take five minutes to breathe. Tomorrow, you might show up at your favorite Zumba class and have to spend half the class hanging out in the back because you just don't have the energy to keep going. Understanding these changes in needs is the key to learning to listen to your body.

Today, I know when to rest. I understand that constantly pushing through doesn't do me any good, but that could all change tomorrow. And when those moments of change occur and I run into obstacles where I can't quite figure out what my body needs, I will turn to my asana practice. I have found that when I put my body in an active state of rest it is easier to tune in and listen to all of its wisdom. Which brings us to our next pose.

CHILD'S POSE (BALASANA)

Child's pose is a resting pose. Most teachers will teach this pose towards the beginning of class, then announce that if at any point you need a break during class you're to come back to this pose.

The first time I ever heard a teacher say this, I thought: *Yeah right, I'm here to work out, why would I take a break? That sounds like I'm giving up.* But taking child's pose isn't giving up or being lazy, it is actually the smartest choice you can make because it indicates that you are truly listening and honoring what your body has to say. If your body needs rest, instead of pushing through you are taking the time to pause and re-collect yourself.

INSTRUCTIONS

To come into child's pose, start on all fours, toes untucked. Bring your big toes together and sep-arate your knees wider than your body. Sit back towards your heels and allow your chest to rest on your thighs. Once your chest is on your thighs, place your forehead on the ground in front of you so that you can fully relax into the pose. Arms can be straight out in front or alongside you.

Now remember, the point here is to listen to your body. If the pose as described above feels terrible, then come out of it and make adjustments. If it feels like your hips are too tight or achy to bring

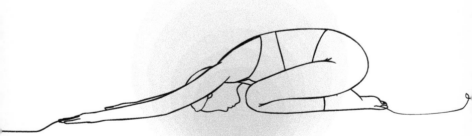

your chest to your thighs, then place a pillow (or five) between your chest and thighs and place more under your forehead so that the weight of your body is fully supported by the pillows and not your body.

If this doesn't feel good, you can try doing this in front of a couch or cushioned chair where you don't have to lean as far forward. You can even take your legs out in front of you.

Regardless of what variation you are in, find a place where you can enter a state of rest but still remain aware of what your body needs. Take a deep breath then relax into the moment so you can continue to **listen to your body.**

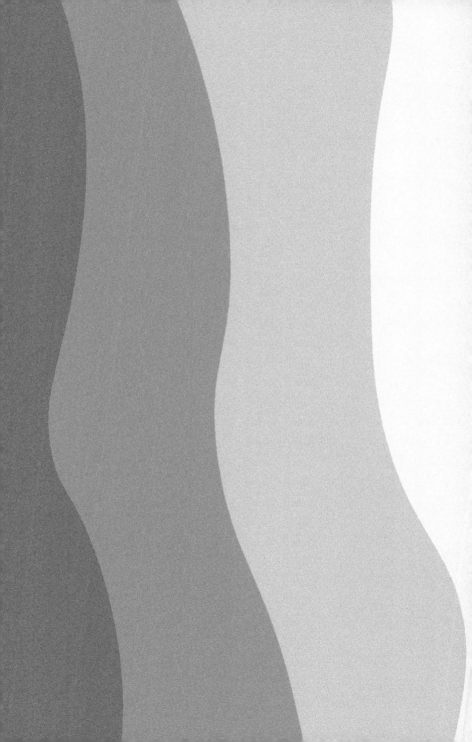

CHAPTER EIGHT

Close Your Eyes

Over the years of teaching, I've developed habits. One is having my students begin every class lying on their backs in savasana with their eyes closed. The students who have been coming to my class or doing yoga on a regular basis quickly close their eyes and settle into the pose. However, there are always one or two people who will close their eyes for a second then pop them open and look around. They'll see others with their eyes closed and close theirs once more—maybe five seconds this time—but inevitably their eyes will pop back open.

At first, I thought these students were uncomfortable because the class was new to them and they didn't know what to expect. Over time, however, I realized that some students never learned to close their eyes for an extended period of time. This made me ask why. As a teacher, I couldn't help but wonder, *Was I doing something wrong?* But afterward, the students would always thank me for a great class, so it had to be something else. *What is it about closing our eyes that's so difficult?* I thought to myself. There are obviously innate human instincts that force us to stay aware of our surroundings. None of us would ever close our eyes in the forest or jungle—hello, lions and tigers and bears! But in a safe space, why is it so hard?

I thought about this for a while and developed a theory: It's difficult to close our eyes because we're constantly worried about what's happening outside of our internal bodies. This is great in the wild, but not so great when we're learning to live in the world and feel better about who we are as human beings. There's a vulnerability to having our eyes closed. In many ways, it's an exposure, an opening up to others. What I concluded was that the students who couldn't keep their eyes closed were worried what others thought about them.

When I first started practicing yoga, I was just like my students. I couldn't close my eyes without worrying that everyone was looking at me, the newbie. Even though all the other students' eyes were supposed to be closed, I kept thinking, *What if they're not? What if they're staring at me?* I was so afraid of what others might think. But now as a teacher, I see a correlation between those who don't close their eyes and how they move their bodies. There's apprehension, and a lack of confidence. In the students who close their eyes, there is an ease. I'm not trying to place judgment on any of this, I'm simply pointing out what I've observed over the years, which adds to my understanding of how our minds and our bodies are connected in more ways than just our health.

When I received my first diagnosis, I was scared to death about what others might think about my new status. My biggest fear then was that no one was going to want to love me because of the disease. I thought, *Who's going to want to take me in sickness and in health, when the sickness is inev-itable?* This fear stayed with me for years, but as my practice progressed and I shared more of my story with the world, I became less and less afraid. I became comfortable with closing my eyes and not worrying about what others thought.

Today, as I deal with the effects of lupus on my body, I find myself returning to this lesson and metaphorically closing my eyes to all those fears. When I have to say no to invites to dinner or can-cel happy hour plans because I'm too fatigued, I close my eyes and don't worry about what my friends think. When I confidently show up to a spin class but realize 20 minutes in that there's no way my body can handle the last 25 minutes, I politely smile at the teacher and leave. I make sure to tell the front desk that it wasn't the teach-er's fault, that she was teaching a good class, but that my legs can't handle the exertion that day and I have to protect my health in order to avoid a bigger flare.

Old me would've pushed right through—no pain, no gain, right? But new me, the one who's had to learn these lessons over and over again, under-stands that pain is a sign from my body telling me to stop and slow down. Being able to close my eyes and look inward and not fret if others think I'm weak or a quitter is how I can make my way through this life with chronic illness.

This is the lesson I want you to learn. I will teach you a pose here, but honestly the biggest thing I want you to take away from this chapter is to learn to close your eyes. I know that might sound silly and you're probably thinking, *I close my eyes every night, it's no big deal.* But have you closed your eyes in public and not worried that others were looking at you or what others thought of you?

That is the real challenge. Try closing your eyes in public spaces. Obviously, don't do this crossing the street—I want you to be safe—but try it in places where people can see you, but won't rob or jump you. I often close my eyes during a pedicure. I'll sit in one of those salons with 20 chairs that's bustling with people, close my eyes, and without fail, when I open them back up the pedicurist always gives me a smile. I've had other patrons look at me like I was strange, but I don't think twice about it anymore. This is the freedom I want for you.

Think about other moments where you can close your eyes and not worry about your safety, but also challenge yourself to be uncomfortable. Can you do it in spin class? At church? Waiting at the DMV—actually don't do that, I don't want you to miss your number being called. Simply find a place where it's awkward to close your eyes and forces you to not care what others think. You can do it for five seconds at a time and work your way up to minutes, maybe hours. If all of that feels uncomfortable, try doing it at home while you're practicing the poses you learn in this book. The more you do it, the easier it will become.

Of course, you can also try this in down dog. The beauty about closing your eyes in down dog, especially when you're in a public class, is that no one can see that your eyes are closed.

DOWN DOG (ADHO MUKHA SVANASANA)

Even if they've never done yoga, down dog is the pose most everyone seems to know. I like to think of down dog as the starting and ending pose that connects all the others.

INSTRUCTIONS

To come into down dog, start on your hands and knees. Place your hands shoulder-distance apart with your fingers spread wide. Press evenly into your fingers so that your weight is distributed throughout your hands and you're not solely

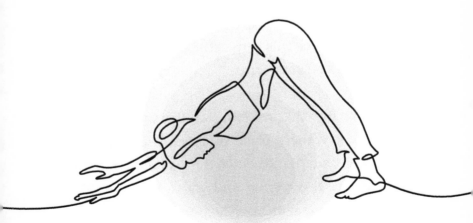

resting on your wrists. Find an external rotation of your arms here—this means that you're slightly twisting your arms out so that the insides of your elbows begin to shine forward.

Once you have this, tuck your toes under so that the balls of your feet are resting on the ground and lift your hips to the sky. Do not be surprised if you can't get your legs fully straight or you can't get your heels to the ground. This may come in time or it might not—either way it's no big deal. The point is that your arms are extended and you're making the effort to move your heels towards the ground and your body is in an inverted V-shape.

If this is too much for your body, that's okay too. You can do down dog at the wall. This will allow you to practice this same shape but take a lot of the weight off your arms.

To come into this version, stand near a wall, facing it. From there place your palms on the wall and walk your hands down the wall until they are parallel to the ground and you're in an upside-down L-shape with your feet on the ground and hands on the wall. If at any point you feel pain or it's too much stretching in your shoulders, then walk your hands back up the wall an inch or two or more and hold where there is no pain.

No matter what version of dog you're holding, close your eyes, take at least five breaths (if not more), and see how that feels. Are you uncomfortable? Are you worrying that someone might walk into the room and see you? Don't judge any of your answers, simply observe. Then watch as your perspective on entering the world with closed eyes begins to change. Open your eyes to the idea that being able to **close your eyes** is a gift.

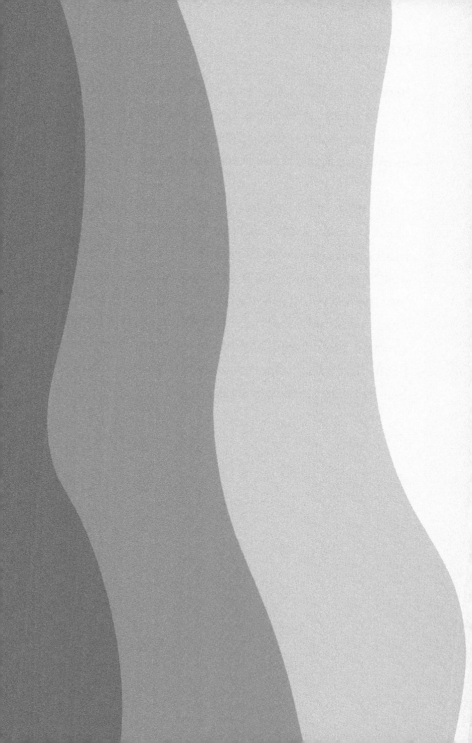

CHAPTER NINE

Stop Comparing Yourself to Others

If there were a nemesis to a life of yoga, it would be comparison. In public classes the tendency is to look at the person next to you or the teacher and think, *If I can't get my body to look exactly like theirs does in the pose, then I'm not doing it right.* I've watched students grunt and force their way into a posture just to be sure they're doing it correctly. But what is correct? Some arbitrary guideline? There's no yoga police stopping you if you do something wrong. There's no one standing there saying you're not as good as the next person. The only right way to do any pose is to do what's right for your body. By playing the comparison game, you only force your body to do something it's not meant to do. The same is true in chronic illness.

Comparison can be our worst enemy. Greater than some of our symptoms, it can take us down and make us feel worse. Comparison is a dead-end effort to make us feel better. Just as it doesn't help to look at the person posing next to me and think they're better than me, comparing my illness to someone else's does me no good either. Thinking, *I could have it worse*, or, *Why am I so much sicker than everyone else with this disease?* doesn't heal my body; it only leads to feelings of inadequacy or superiority. The comparison game puts us at odds with fellow compatriots, those who are often the only ones who understand what we're going through.

When I was first diagnosed with MS, I spent hours on the internet searching for answers. In my search, I stumbled upon several chat rooms filled with other MS patients. In these rooms, I found myself spiraling until three or four in the morning, reading about all the possible things that could happen to me. These rooms were not positive places. People weren't happy. Instead, they were playing a game of comparison. Someone would write about their annoying or devastating symptom and people wouldn't share how they dealt with it personally and offer sound and caring advice. Instead, they would compound on the person's original problem. If someone had numbness in their hands, then the next person had it in their hands and arms, and the next person had it in their hands, arms, and torso. They were not only comparing themselves but also trying to one-up each other. While I never commented on any of the chats, I certainly got swept into the game of comparison and it completely freaked me out. Reading about all these possibilities had me worried that A) maybe I didn't belong with the other MS patients because I didn't have it bad enough yet, and B) all of these horrible symptoms were going to happen to my body one day. While some or all of those thoughts might have been true, none of them helped my current state.

Often, comparison can be worse than the symptoms. Every time I compare myself and my health to others, I always feel worse. I have yet to meet a person who's played the comparison game and come out on top. We all have our own stories and our own health to manage, and trying to enter someone else's story through comparison is futile—we will never become the star. There will always be differences between all of us on this planet. We will be sicker, healthier, sadder, happier than others. This is a fact of life but one we can deal with through our practice.

During my time in the chat rooms playing the comparison game, my only saving grace was that I was going to a yoga class every day. Those classes saved me. When I would step onto my mat, I would forget about everything I'd read because I could only focus on where and how my body was moving in that moment. I had no time to compare myself to others or worry about the future of my health. At that point I had been practicing for nearly two years and could tune out the other students around me. I was so inwardly focused that I didn't have the time or the wherewithal to compare myself to anyone around me. In those hours on my mat, I learned that focus was the perfect antidote to comparison. It's really hard to balance on one leg if you're constantly darting your eyes all over the room. The same is true in our lives.

If you can focus on one singular point—whether it's your body, or your breath, or a spot on the wall—you don't have the mental capacity to compare. When you can bring your focus back to something outside yourself, you can find balance and not get bogged down by others' stories.

The perfect pose to begin working on focus, or the concept of dharana, is side plank.

SIDE PLANK (VASISTHASANA)

The side plank is an introduction to balance in the physical sense. This can be a physically challenging pose, but do not fret. I am going to give you options so that no matter what state your body is in, you can form this shape in one way or another. Please don't go on Instagram or Google and look for the "perfect" way to do this pose. I want you to look inward and find a shape with your body where you have to work to find balance and focus on one singular thing.

INSTRUCTIONS

Start on your hands and knees. Move your right hand forward about six inches. Lean into your right hand and shift your weight onto your right knee and shin. Turn your torso so that your hips are stacked. Extend your left leg so your left foot remains on the ground to help you balance. Your right hand, right knee, and left foot should all be in one line. Your weight should be in your right hand and your right shin and it should feel like

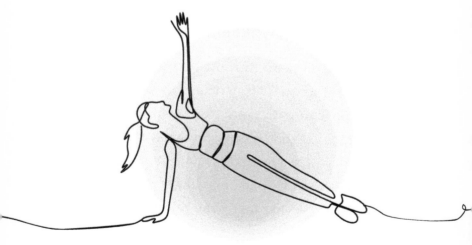

you're leaning against a wall. In fact, you can do this next to a wall so that you can lean back against it to help you balance. Extend your left arm straight to the sky so that it stacks directly above your right arm. Hold here for five breaths. Repeat on the other side.

To come into another version that might challenge your balance even more, sit on your right hip and place your right hand firmly on the ground. Extend your legs and stack both your feet on top of one another. Flex through your feet, lift your hips so that they're in line with your shoulder. Your body should be in one straight line. It should look like you're a standing person but just tilted onto the ground.

Whatever version you're in remember to keep the focus on the pose and **stop comparing yourself to others.**

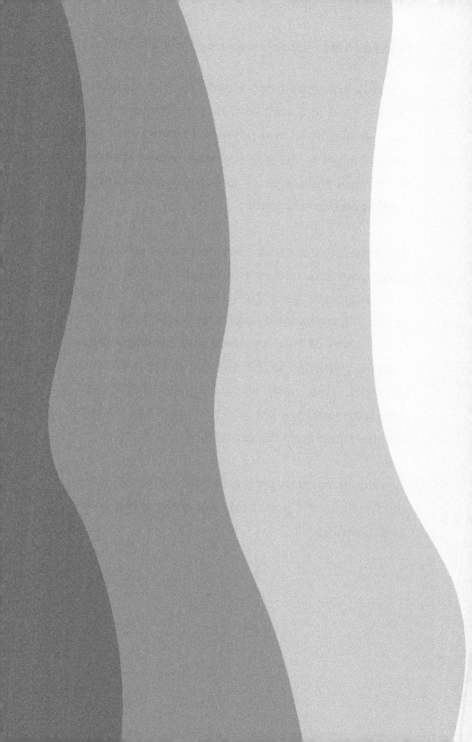

CHAPTER **TEN**

Don't Worry, Be

I used to fear going to sleep. My fear wasn't the kind of fear I had when I was young, worrying about the dark, the boogeyman, or the shadow in the corner. Instead, my fear was that I would wake up and not be able to walk.

I feared that one day all the possible symptoms of MS would hit me overnight and I'd wake to find that the world as I knew it was over. That I could no longer walk, practice yoga, bike. I lived with this deep-seated anxiety that everything that could go wrong would go wrong in the middle of the night. So, I barely slept. Instead, I would watch overly dramatized medical shows on TV until the wee hours of the morning. Then, around 4 a.m., I would finally drift off to sleep—not because I wanted to, but because my body forced me to. I would wake, and when I found that nothing drastic happened to my physical body overnight, I would say a little prayer of thanks and try to go about my day. But inevitably, because of the lack of sleep, I would need a nap in the afternoon. Those naps were my only real sleep during that time. I felt safe in these naps because I had convinced myself that napping during the day was fine because the sun was still out and obviously nothing bad ever happens during the day—right?

I spent two years living like this—in complete and utter fear of the dark. The worry overtook me and I didn't know how to live the way I once had before—carefree. Looking back now, I can see it was a fear of the unknown.

The unknown is the scariest of beasts when you're dealing with chronic illness, especially when you've had symptoms that are devastating, go away, then threaten to return. One of my friends said it well when she stated that it's often harder to live with the unknown and the fears of the future than it is to deal with the symptoms of the disease. The mental game is rough. I agree with her. Sometimes it's easier to power through the pain, or take a day off, or find pharmaceutical relief. With the mental aspect, there is no real escape.

I've been dealing with disease since 2007, and I still worry that the MS will render me immobile. I also live in fear that the pleurisy in my lungs that resulted from the lupus is going to come back and I'll be sidelined from most physical activities again. I worry that the lupus will attack my vital organs, that the fatigue will affect my writing. I worry that I might die young. I worry that I'll never have kids. I worry about anything and everything. And if I let them, these fears can overtake my days.

The good news is that I've learned to see that everything is cyclical and the longer I keep living the more some of these thoughts dissipate.

With MS, I no longer worry that I'm going to wake up one morning and not be able to walk. Sure, I still live with the idea that one day my legs, my arms, my body will fail me, but as time passes and the mornings that I wake up unchanged go from just a few days to years, I start to believe that I will be okay. That maybe, for now, I've escaped the horrible wrath of MS that I had created in my head.

I now see that my worrying was just a waste of time, because nothing happens overnight with these chronic illnesses. That's not how they work. They progress slowly.

I know this thanks to lupus. The disease's progress was a gradual trickle—going from symptoms I could ignore to symptoms that were unbearable. First the bone pain set in. Then the fatigue had me constantly napping, exhausted after walking a flight of two stairs. Then my heart faltered, and my lungs filled with fluid. I could barely breathe, and I no longer tolerated exercise. Then my writing suffered, and my editors thought I lost my ability to write. Bit by bit, everything was taken away from me. But because everything happened so slowly, I didn't have time to worry because I was too busy dealing with the present symptoms.

Instead, I only had the capacity to deal with what was right in front of me. I leaned on my yoga practice; it taught me that leaning into the moment was the way to the other side.

The present was a gift once more. Fearing the dark would take me nowhere. Relinquishing control over my future, however, helped me stay in the moment. Letting go and letting god, as the concept of isvara pranidhana teaches, was how I stopped worrying. It wasn't easy getting here, and I will be the first to tell you that it's not always easy to maintain, either. I still fall back into cycles of worry, but when I do now, I immediately turn to asanas. The physical part of yoga helps me to break the cycle.

One of the greatest aspects about asanas is that they can act as a guide back to the present.

When we challenge our physical bodies in a way that requires all our faculties, then we don't have time to worry about the future or fret about the past. All we can do is stay present in the moment and pay attention to what our bodies are doing in the here and now (similar to how it's easier to deal with symptoms because they are in the moment and banging on our front door). One of the biggest benefits of doing a challenging physical pose is that it forces you to pay close attention. This does not mean that you need to replicate some super-hard pose you saw in a magazine. Instead it means finding the physical activity that pushes your current limits. Some days for me, that challenge is simply taking a shower. Other days, I require a long walk or a flow through a few yoga poses. No matter what my capabilities of that day are, movement is key.

Movement in this sense means to go with the flow. Do not resist when your body asks you to push further and don't force it when it's telling you to just chill. Like the instructions for getting caught in a riptide say, "Do not panic, don't try to swim against the current." Your job when it comes to honoring your body and escaping the cycle of worry is to go with the flow. When you fight against nature, you make everything harder. When you flow with nature, you make it easier.

One of my favorite short flows is a half sun salute. As long as I'm not having a high pain day, this is usually something I can do to clear my mind of the worries and bring me back to the present. If you're having a high pain day or fatigue has set in, you probably won't need this flow because your own symptoms act as a reminder to stay present. But if you do need them, use this set of poses to focus your mind on the moment.

MOUNTAIN POSE (TADASANA) AND HALF SUN SALUTE (ARDHA SURYA NAMASKAR)

Mountain pose is the first most challenging pose and the foundation for everything else. It might look like you're just standing up straight, but it is so much more. Placing your body into a position that requires subtle movements of the muscles and concentration forces you to sit in the present.

The half sun salute is a way to move your body that forces you to pay attention to the moment, because not only do you have to focus on your body but also your breath.

INSTRUCTIONS

For mountain pose, stand with your feet parallel. They can be hips' width apart or you can have your big toes touching with your heels slightly apart. Relax your shoulders and let your arms hang heavy alongside you. Turn your palms to face directly in front of you. Rock slightly forward and back so that you can find a place where your weight is distributed evenly through your feet. Flex your thigh muscles and spin them inwards towards the back of the room. Although it'll appear as if you're simply standing, every muscle in your body should be engaged in some way.

If you can't stand today (and I mean physically can't stand up, not *I can't stand this today*), you can do this lying on your back with your feet against a wall. You can still engage all the same muscles, even if you're lying on your back.

To move through a half sun salute, as you inhale circle your arms up overheard. Keep your arms as straight as possible. If you can keep your elbows straight, touch your palms together; otherwise keep them shoulder width apart. As you exhale, circle your arms back down to your sides. (This whole set of arm movements does not have to be done standing and can easily be done in a seated or even supine position.)

Repeat this circling motion of the arms five times. Inhale reach your arms overhead, exhale draw them to your sides. On the fifth time, draw your hands to your chest, exhale, and bend at the waist to fold all the way forward. On an inhale, raise your torso halfway, slide your hands up your shins, and open your chest. Imagine that

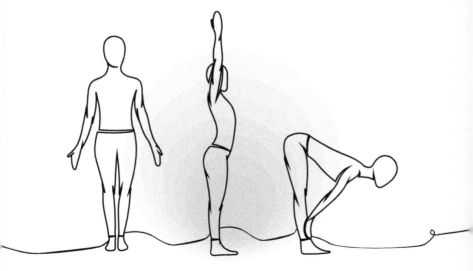

you are pulling something through the middle of your heart center. Exhale and fold all the way forward again, and as you inhale circle your arms out to the side and all the way up as you come to stand with arms overhead. Exhale draw your hands down in front of your chest in prayer position. You can repeat this cycle as many times as you need to draw your focus back to the present so that you **don't worry,** and just **be.**

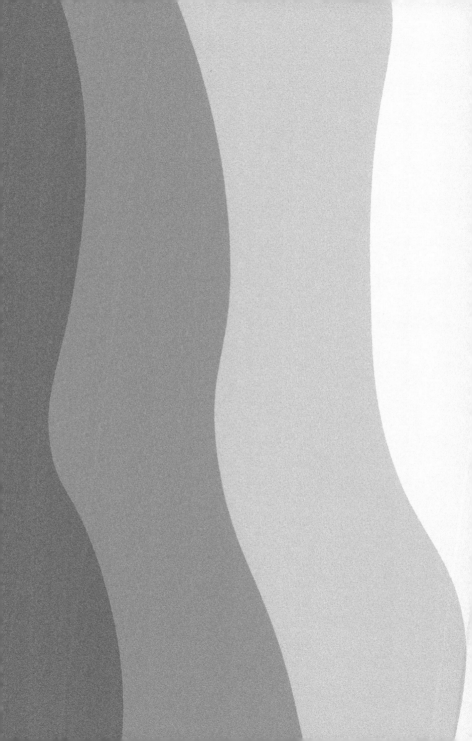

CHAPTER ELEVEN

You Are Not Alone

Living with chronic illness can be isolating, because no one—unless they're living it too—fully understands. I don't know about you, but when people ask me how I'm doing, it's often a lot easier to say "fine" instead of going into the full details of how I'm really feeling that day. No one wants to hear that I woke up with excruciating pain in my legs, and I haven't showered because that required too much energy, and now I really just want to watch TV, but I'm here working because I need the money to pay for my prescriptions. They want to hear that I'm doing "just fine." So, I ignore the teachings of satya and power through with no honesty.

But living on this fine line of trying to pretend we're okay and asking for help can be isolating. We may protect ourselves from the hurt that comes with the vulnerability of sharing our struggles, but we also end up shielding ourselves from any help others might offer.

In that way, living with an invisible illness is a blessing and a curse. On the one hand, we don't have to tell anyone what we're going through if we don't want to. Yet, on the other hand, it's often hard for others to understand what we're going through because we don't look sick. In that case, secrets then become easier to deal with than the disease itself, so we turn to them.

For eight years, only my closest friends and family knew I was living with MS. I hid it because I was ashamed and worried that others would see me differently. The last thing I wanted was to feel like an outsider, like I was different, or that I no longer belonged. So I kept everything hidden and maintained the façade that I was perfectly fine. In reality, however, I was far from fine. I needed help. But since I had hidden my struggles, no one knew I needed support. My pretending was a double-edged sword: It made me feel less different, but it also isolated me from others. I believed I was in this fight alone. It wasn't until I started writing about my experiences with chronic illness that I began to see that I was not on this journey solo.

When my memoir, *Love Sick*, was published, most people didn't know I had been dealing with MS. I created a separate Instagram account that didn't include any of my friends. Instead, I made it my safe space to share my story. There, I connected with so many other men and women who were also dealing with MS and other chronic illnesses. They became my tribe and they made me feel less alone.

Connecting with my tribe reiterated the truth that none of us are in this world by ourselves. At times, it may feel like we are, but there is always someone who has had similar experiences. We might have to search online, seek help from doctors or nurses, find groups of fellow chronically living folks on social media, or ask for a referral to a therapist. No matter what, though, we can find what we're looking for if we stand strong in our truth. Living with a chronic illness is not easy, and we are not meant to do this alone.

Yoga means "union," and that can translate not just to our bodies and our minds, but to others as well. It's meant to serve as a reminder that we are all in this together, both literally and figuratively. I remember one of the classes I attended when I first began practicing. After a nice flow, our teacher had us move into a circle. You know, the kind you make when you're in elementary school. When we had moved into a nice circle shape, she announced that we would be practicing tree pose. Tree pose is a balancing pose where you stand on one leg and place the other foot on the inside of the balancing leg. It's one of those poses that looks simple but can be quite challenging, especially if your balance is off that day.

Once we were in the circle the teacher instructed us to place our right hand on the shoulder of the person to the right of us and our left hand on the small of the back of the person to the left of us. Then we each lifted our left leg off the ground and placed it on the inside of our right leg. We were all in tree pose, yet we were all fully supported because we literally had each others' backs.

Since that day, I've loved tree pose, not only because it challenges my balance, but because it serves as a literal and metaphorical reminder that we are not alone. In fact, in nature trees are actually connected to one another. Scientists have discovered that trees rely on each other to survive. They are not solitary strong beings holding their own in the forest, instead they are holding themselves up with the help of each other. We can do the same.

By practicing tree pose, we can remind ourselves that we are all in this together. As you move through this pose, think about the people around the world who might be practicing it as well. Think about other readers who are reading this too, other patients like you, standing strong together.

TREE POSE (VRKSASANA)

Tree pose is a balancing pose, but it can be modified for any body. Maybe you can't balance today, but maybe you can place your body in the shape of a tree in some form to remind yourself that you are a part of an entire network of beings on this planet, and we are looking out for you.

INSTRUCTIONS

If your balance is currently off, I suggest you stand next to a chair, a wall, or a desk, or even a friend to help you so that you don't fall.

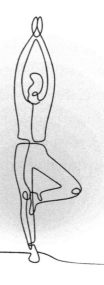

To begin, stand up tall in mountain pose (page 129). Once you feel steady here, raise your right or left foot and gently place it on the inside of your opposite leg. You can place it as low as the ankle or as high as the inner thigh, but avoid placing it directly on the inside of the knee.

Once you have your balance, move your hands to prayer position or overhead. If you really want to challenge yourself, close your eyes. Repeat on the other side.

As you stand strong in this pose, let it serve as a reminder that **you are not alone.**

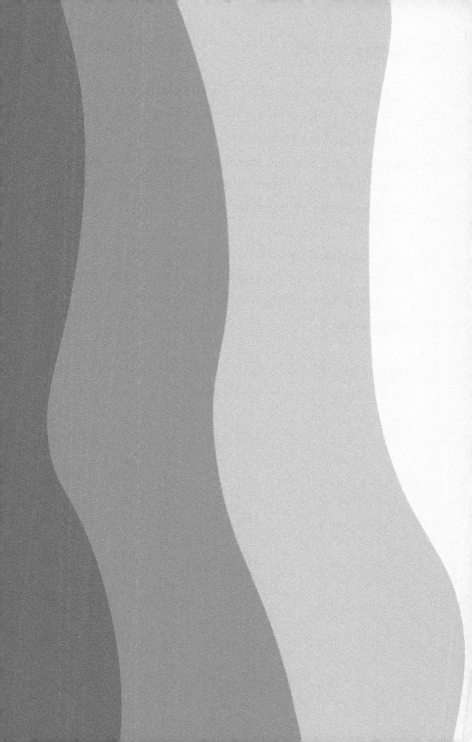

CHAPTER TWELVE
Just Say No

I grew up in the Reagan "Just Say No" era, so saying no was ingrained in me. I learned not to take drugs—they would fry my brains like an egg on a skillet. But what I didn't learn was how to say no to the things that waste my energy (hello, brahmacharya). If I could go back, I would teach myself those skills. I would teach myself that I don't always have to go full-out and embrace all of life with a no pain, no gain attitude. Instead, I would teach myself the principle of asteya—to not steal. I would teach my younger self not to steal from my energy stores, nor allow someone else to. Saying no isn't about letting someone down, or risking them saying something that's not kind; it's about protecting yourself.

"I'm tired too" is what everyone seems to say when you tell them you're tired. Except your tired looks nothing like their tired. Your tired is legit fatigue. Your tired is the kind of tired that you see at the end of marathons, where competitors have to crawl over the finish line, only you just walked upstairs. Your tired makes the thought of getting out of bed sound exhausting. Your tired keeps you from showering for days. Your tired makes everything feel impossible.

My fiancé and I actually got into a fight over this kind of tired once. We had just moved into a new house and I was exhausted from the day of hauling boxes and directing movers. I had used every ounce of energy I had in my ill body. By the time the movers had gone, I told him I was showering and going to bed. He said he wanted to order dinner. "I'm fine," I said, meaning that I didn't want to eat, but he took it as a passive aggressive way of saying I can't deal with this anymore (moving always brings out the best in all of us!). When I got out of the shower, he hadn't yet ordered his dinner. I asked why and he said he was waiting for me. I reiterated that I didn't want anything. "I'm tired," I said.

"Well, that's weird," he said. "We always eat together." I realized my words didn't properly communicate my current mental and physical state. I tried again.

"I am so fatigued and exhausted that the thought of having to chew my dinner sounds like too much," I said. "I don't think I can do it." He looked at me in horror, but he understood. It was a good lesson and reminder that my definition of tired and a healthy person's definition of tired are vastly different.

So often the world wants us to get better. People will help us with our initial diagnosis, but then they forget that this thing doesn't go away. I don't blame them. Before I was "sick," I thought the same thing. Why can't someone just get better? I now know that that's not always possible and I understand that sometimes you have to be direct and explicit when it comes to your illness. We can't rely on others to figure it out. It's up to us to explain to others how we truly feel. It's up to us to come back to satya and be honest.

When everything seems, feels, and actually is exhausting, I know it's far easier to say we're tired instead of fully explaining. Sometimes, it's easier to push through than have to tell someone that we're on the brink of being out of energy stores or that we're so close to flaring it's not even funny. It's easier to say, "I'll be fine," even when we know it's not true.

Often, I push through not because I feel good, but because I don't want to hear someone say, "I'm tired too" or, "It's just a couple of blocks, you can totally walk there." So, instead I say okay, and do what I'm told. But in the long run, I end up hurting myself because I simply can't say no.

I know that saying no is the best choice for me in many of these moments, yet this yogic philosophy of not stealing energy is one that takes practice and time to learn. Our bodies and their needs are constantly changing from day to day, and it's hard to know when we're stealing energy from one day to the next. However, in the long run, I know that this is a game of saying no and saying yes at all the right times, or simply learning to parse out my stores of energy as I go through the day.

When I first started to learn this concept, I thought about my yoga teachers who would say, "You can do anything for 30 seconds." In that arena the 30-second note was meant to say that you can push through. But now when I remember this I think, *This is what I can handle. I can do something for 30 seconds. I don't have to push myself to the limits. I can simply do something for 30 seconds or less.* Giving myself the permission to do something for 30 seconds a day takes off all the pressure. I no longer have to be upset about all the things I lost, the things the diseases took away from me. Instead, I can run my own mini-marathons and when I say marathon, I mean anything that is done to improve my state of being. This can be anything from brushing my teeth, to taking a walk, to sitting up in bed and walking to the couch. By acknowledging that I don't have to run for hours or even clean the house for an hour, I can give myself permission that all the work I do doesn't have to be full-out pedal to the metal. I can take things slow. Learning to say no helps you recognize that you don't have to do anything crazy to work on your health. What a relief! It gives you the permission to not change everything all at once. I don't have to change my diet or meal prep for the week, or get on a strict weight training regimen, or even do yoga every day to feel better. I can improve my health 30 seconds at a time.

You can do this too. It doesn't have to be anything crazy. It can literally be taking three deep breaths. Doing something to prove to yourself that you can do anything for that short amount of time will help you learn to slow down and not go all-out. When you feel overwhelmed, set your timer on your phone for 30 seconds then do something physical for that time. Whether it's standing in tree, holding a side plank, resting in child's pose, or closing your eyes and putting your head on your desk. Putting a 30-second limit on activities proves that anything is possible without draining yourself, even if it's just sitting in a chair.

CHAIR POSE (UTKATASANA)

Easing into chair pose stands as a reminder that though life may be difficult, you can sit through all of it. In its traditional expression, chair pose builds and requires strength in your thighs and core plus good balance. However, for our purposes, I want you to look at chair pose as a reminder that we can ease ourselves into something for 30 seconds at a time without stealing all of our energy.

INSTRUCTIONS

Stand in mountain pose (page 129). Bend your knees and move your hips down and back as if you're sitting in a chair. Arms can remain alongside you or you can extend them to the sky. Once you've bent your knees shift your weight into your heels so that if you look down you can see your toes.

The traditional expression of this pose can be quite draining, which we don't want, so here are a few options. To put you in the same shape but not require all of the energy, find a chair, sit on the edge with your feet firmly planted on the ground.

Squeeze your glutes together (i.e., clench your butt cheeks) and lift your arms overhead. Continue to breathe. Do this for 30 seconds.

If that's too much, lie on your back with your feet against the wall and your knees bent. Press into your feet and extend your arms over head. If this is too much work for you today, then stack a bunch

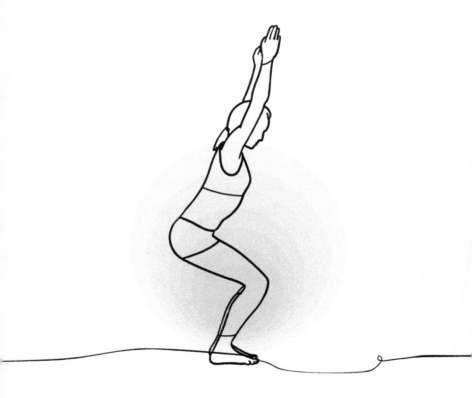

of pillows under your calves to help support the weight of your legs.

Find a shape that works for you and your current energy stores and **just say no** to whatever doesn't work for you!

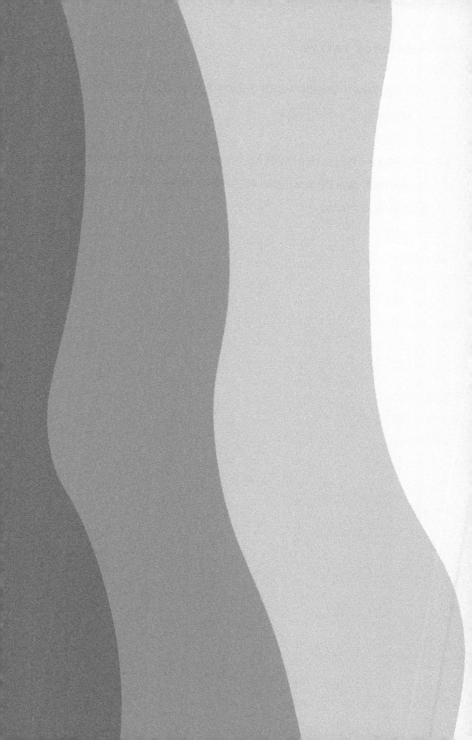

CHAPTER THIRTEEN

Stop Playing by the Rules

Medicine is not an exact science. There are some absolutes, but most of the time it is a guessing game of trial and error, a reliance on theories that have been proven but will most likely be unproven one day. We all know this. There are no concrete answers to our conditions.

There are no hard and fast rules when it comes to medicine and our health. We can feel amazing one day and end up in a hospital bed the next. We can't play by the rules because they are ever changing. When I first developed pleurisy and my lungs were inflamed, getting dressed in the morning wiped me out. Even though the drugs were helping, they weren't perfect. When I asked my doctor whether there were other solutions, he couldn't give me a concrete answer. There were things I could try, but there was no trial-and-tested protocol to follow. The same is true for your yoga practice. It is your practice, not mine or anyone else's.

When I first started practicing yoga, I was the geeky student who paid attention to every cue and instruction. I strived to put my body in the "correct" position every time. I believed there was one way to do each pose, and I hadn't mastered anything until a teacher stopped adjusting me.

What I now know through self-study (svadhyaya) is that there is no correct way to do a pose. In fact, my body is not even physically capable of following the "right" way in many positions. But this is okay. This is the way it's supposed to be.

As you move forward with your yoga practice, please remember there are no rules. Your practice is your practice. There is no correct way to do anything—the poses, the self-study, the meditation, the breathing. The only correct way is the way that works for you in the moment.

This is why there is no pose here. The only "pose" I want to give you is to be free.

BE FREE

To be free is to act without constraint or worry or desire. It is to truly live in the present moment. This is the most important pose of the entire practice.

INSTRUCTIONS

Throughout this book, I have laid out poses and taught you philosophies, but my way is not the only way. I want you to find your way. Find a place where you feel comfortable simply being—whether that's in bed, on the couch, in a chair, or standing in an open space.

Now close your eyes and scan your body. How does it feel in this moment? What does it need? What do you feel like doing? Napping? Skipping? Dancing? Stretching? Doing down dog? Start moving with no goal or purpose. Simply move because it feels good in that moment. Do what feels right. Be free and **stop playing by the rules.**

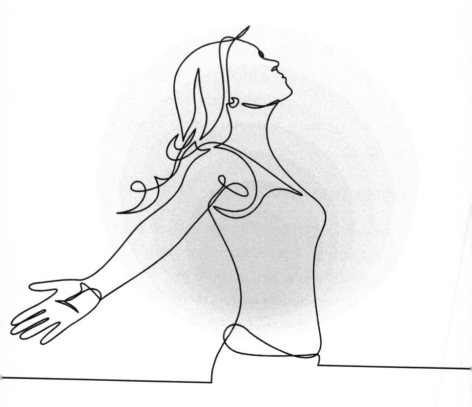

CHAPTER FOURTEEN
Surrender to What Is

When we're newly diagnosed, we want answers. We want to know: Why? How? What can we do to fix it? But some questions don't have answers and this is where we become stuck. It's difficult to accept the unknown. As humans, the need for an explanation is great. When we don't get answers, we make up stories and form theories of why we feel the way we do—and then we take these theories as fact. I ate gluten, that's why my bones hurt. I drank wine, that's why I'm fatigued. I worked out too much, that's why I'm in pain. I should only eat raw vegetables if I want to heal.

We do our best to explain the way we feel, regardless of whether our theories are backed by science or recommended by our doctors. Even though we know that so much of living with chronic illness is learning to live with its unpredictability, we try to predict it all. When I was diagnosed with lupus, I believed that the answers to all my problems could be found in my diet. I did a lot of research and was encouraged by so many claims by people who no longer had evidence of disease or who had reversed their disease through diet.

Believing I was 100 percent responsible for my well-being, I dived headfirst into changing my diet. I followed all these different diets that claimed to cure and aid in symptom relief of autoimmune diseases—the Autoimmune Protocol, Wahls Protocol, Dr. Gundry's Plant Paradox, Dr. Fuhrman's Nutritarian diet. Clean eating. Fasting. I changed so much about my diet, but none of it made a huge difference. Yet, I felt wholeheartedly that I could fix my disease. But this is where the problem lies in trying to fix everything yourself. When things go wrong or don't improve, you are now at fault. When I had bad days or weeks, I felt responsible for all the aches and pains. Since I'd taken it upon myself to cure the diseases by my alternative, Google-hacked methods, I felt responsible when they didn't work. When I had bad days, it was now my fault. When my health didn't improve, I was to blame. No longer were bad days simply chalked up to the fact that I have lupus and MS; they were chalked up to that sugar-laden, gluten-filled slice of cake I ate the night before.

This pattern of self-blame repeated itself for nearly a year. Now not only were the symptoms my fault, the disease was my fault too. I had caused all of it. I truly believed that anything and everything I did or didn't do would affect my outcome. I was trapped in a spiral of believing that I had complete control. But the truth is I had no control. I have two highly unpredictable and incurable diseases. This is fact. No amount of healthy eating will ever cure me. No amount of Googling will allow me to rise out of bed every single morning for the rest of my life with boundless energy. These were hard truths I had to sit with. Despite the fact that I so desperately wanted to change the course of my health on my own, I had to accept my reality.

When I realized this, I turned back to yoga to practice satya (or truth) and decided to surrender to the truths of the disease.

The truth is MS can destroy the protective coating on your nerves, causing a variety of symptoms from numbness and blindness to spasticity and incontinence and more. No one can predict how it will affect any individual. There are some drugs to slow the progression and others for varying symptoms, but the one way to know how it will affect you as an individual is to continue to live through it. The truth with lupus is that your immune system can decide to attack any part of your body at any point in time. It can cause kidney failure, heart disease, heart attack, and stroke. It can cause fatigue and joint pain. It can do anything it wants, really. There are several drugs that can control its effects and slow the disease process, but there is no absolute.

The truth with both diseases is that they are life altering. But life altering doesn't mean life ending. My life is not over. There are many things I can do, and I can choose to see the good in that. I can do my best and honor my body's limitations. I can acknowledge that there will be good days *and* bad days. I can write this book. I can cultivate close relationships with family and friends. I can pursue my dreams. I can adjust to my reality and my new normal. I can practice gratitude for all of these things.

I can give thanks. I can choose to see the beauty in all that I've been through. It doesn't mean that it's been easy, but it does mean that I've changed into someone I really love and appreciate. I can acknowledge my self-actualization as one of my greatest life accomplishments.

I had a therapist once tell me that most people spend their lives looking for a purpose, and that often, people who experience life-altering diagnoses find their purposes much sooner than others. I don't know that I can clearly articulate what my purpose is, but perhaps it's putting this message out into the world. I do know, however, that I've reached a point of contentment (santosha), and a feeling that I can let go and let it be. I am in the ultimate now—the isvara pranidhana.

In yoga, they tell you to surrender into the pose, which means to let go of control. Your body knows where it needs to go. Your body will stop you from moving into a place of harm. Your body will support you when your muscles start to quiver, and it will tell you when it's time to take a break. But if you keep forcing it and overriding its own natural knowledge, you will start to cause harm. You will feel responsible for the things that are 100 percent out of your control. You will stress yourself out. If you can slow down and remind yourself to surrender to what is, you might just learn to open yourself up to a world of possibility that isn't clouded by worry or control. You might be able to find gratitude for everything life has thrown at you.

This won't be easy, but you can take it one step at a time. Yoga is a practice. Maybe today you can only surrender to what is within a space of five minutes. Maybe tomorrow, you'll surrender to the fact that some days you won't have the energy to complete your entire to-do list. Perhaps the next day, you'll surrender to a little more. Bit by bit, you will relinquish more and more of your desire to control everything. You will be able to lie gently on your back, close your eyes, be vulnerable, and accept that you have no control. You will surrender to what is.

SAVASANA

At the beginning of the book, we used savasana as a way to check in with ourselves and start our day in an informed manner. Now, when we lie here at the end of our day or our practice, we can use savasana as a place to learn to surrender. When we bring our thoughts back to the body, we can now check in—but not to inform how we will go about our day, but to see how we can let go of all we've experienced over the day. In the letting go, we can find the moments of bliss.

INSTRUCTIONS

In fourth grade, my teacher, Ms. Vicelli, led our class through the exact same exercise I'm about to teach you. Even at nine years old I reveled in the feeling of complete surrender. I knew that she had taught us something special. This exercise is something that I have used throughout my entire life. Something that I come back to now at 40 years old, ready to use to face whatever the universe decides to throw my way. This is what I want to leave you with.

Lie on your back in a comfortable position where you are in the least amount of pain possible. From there, you will go into the exercise of surrender.

STEPS TO SURRENDER

To surrender, move through your entire body, tensing each muscle then relaxing it.

First curl your feet into themselves. Clench the muscles of your toes and your soles as hard as you can. Hold for five seconds then relax.

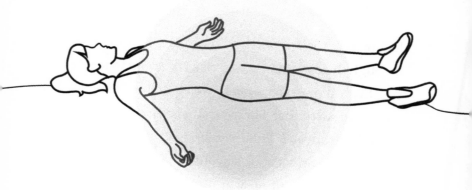

Now move to your calves. Tighten those muscles, hold for five seconds then relax.

Now go to your thighs and repeat the same pattern. Continue doing this pattern as you make your way up your body to your glutes/butt, then stomach, then chest. Hands, then forearms and biceps. Shoulders, neck, and face.

Once you've tightened and relaxed every muscle in your body take a deep breath in through your nose and open your mouth and sigh it out.

You are now in a place of surrender. Stay here and breathe for as long as you need to **surrender to what is.**

CHAPTER FIFTEEN
Pull It Together

In the same way that you've had to pull together your charts, your symptoms, your test results, and various doctors' opinions, you can also pull together everything you learned here in this book to help you continue with your yoga practice.

While each chapter focused solely on one pose and a philosophy, you can also put them into one longer sequence that you can do when your body allows. Remember, the most important thing to do in any asana practice is listen to your body. Do not push past your limits. Don't try to force anything. Surrender to what is and remember that every day your limits and your capabilities will change. Don't get down on yourself if today's not the day where you can go a little longer than 30 seconds, just accept who you are in the moment and embrace it.

SEQUENCE

Savasana (page 53): As you begin your practice, remember to **be here now.** Use this moment to check in with your body. How does it feel? What does it need? What should you avoid?

Forward fold (page 66): **Give yourself props** for showing up and doing this sequence. As you fold forward, remember that props—whether they be words or physical objects—are the smart choice to help you ease into each pose.

Easy pose with twists (page 77 & 81): Remember that there is no shortcut to a yoga practice or chronic illness. **Slow down and embrace the beginner within.** Allow yourself the time to move through all the stages of grief.

Cat/cow (page 91): No matter how many times you think about these philosophies or move through these poses, remember that **practice makes life.** By paying attention and staying aware of how your body feels as you move, and how it reacts to your daily life, you can learn what is best for you.

Child's pose (page 101): Take a moment to pause and reflect. Child's pose is a reminder to not just listen to your needs, but to also act upon them. Despite what outside forces might say, the idea of no pain, no gain should be eliminated from your thought process. Now is the time to **listen to your body,** not ignore it.

Down dog (page 111): Settle into this pose, **close your eyes,** and remind yourself that worrying about what others think will get you nowhere. Stand strong in who you are at your very core.

Side plank (page 120): Use this balancing pose to find focus so that you can **stop comparing your-self to others.** Remember that in the comparison game, no one wins.

Mountain pose/half sun salute (page 131): When you find your mind wandering, fretting about the past, and worrying about the future, come back to the moment. Use your breath and movement to stay present. Your mantra here is **don't worry, be.**

Tree (page 140): There is an entire forest out there supporting you in your every move. Lean on others for support, share your story in solidarity, and remember that **you are not alone.**

Chair (page 150): You might struggle here, you might feel the burn in your thighs, but there is nothing set in stone saying you have to hold this pose forever. You can sit down, then stand right back up. You can sit in an actual chair. The power is yours. If you are wasting too much energy on the poses, on pleasing others, or on working harder and you have nothing left to give, remind yourself that it's okay to **just say no.**

Be free: If today is not the day for all of these poses or any of these poses, remember that the most important pose, the most important part of this entire practice is to move with wild abandon and **stop playing by the rules.**

Savasana (page 166): When you've had enough, when you're ready to relax, when you're ready to embrace all that lies ahead of you, find a place of comfort where you can close your eyes and completely let go. **Surrender to what is.**

CONCLUSION
Namaste

When I first started yoga, I kept hearing practitioners and teachers talk about taking the lessons learned on the mat into the world. I practiced nearly every day for two years before I fully understood what that meant. I didn't understand the philosophy, or the lessons, or that holding the poses is only a means to an end. I didn't know then that the real yoga, the thing that will change your life, is the yoga that teaches patience, the ability to surrender and focus on what matters. The real yoga is being able to be present to the here and now.

Someone asked me once: "What is the biggest difference between today and the days I was first diagnosed?" If I could choose one word to describe the difference between now and the day the doctors told me I had these illnesses, it would be *aware*. My awareness didn't happen overnight, but living with such unpredictable diseases makes you see the world through a different lens. It showed me how to live in a new way. It showed me that a life with chronic illness means I am now more aware of my body—when it needs to rest, when I need to push it, when I need to adjust my diet or workouts or work schedule.

Living with chronic illness made me aware that this is the only body I get, and its abilities are ever changing, so I should appreciate every moment that I can do the things I enjoy. I am now more aware of the time I spend doing the things I love, and the time I spend on the things I have to do to pay bills.

I am aware that everything could change tomorrow, so I do my best to stay present. I am aware that I am not alone, that we are all facing unseen battles, whether it's rheumatoid arthritis, cancer, lupus, or something else, and I operate with a different sense of compassion. I am aware that saying yes to new things is better than saying no and wondering what would've happened. I am aware that when I say yes, I need to do it from a place of understanding my body.

I am fully aware that I have limitations and it's up to me to set boundaries. I am aware that the only constant in this world is change and I try to embrace it. I am aware that I am powerful because I have been through challenges that have shaped me into a better version of myself.

I am now aware that I was learning yoga's philosophies and edicts all along. The practice of yoga didn't change my fundamental being; it simply gave me a structure to apply changes to my life. It opened me up to a world of possibility and a tribe of others who understand my struggles. Yoga created a community when I needed one most. You are now part of that community, and for that I am grateful. Together, we can support each other in this crazy world of disease—and I know we will.

At the end of every traditional yoga class, it is common to bow your head and say "namaste." The word can be translated as, "The divine light in me salutes the divine light in you." Meaning, I honor the part of you that makes me the same as you. As a fellow chronic illness superstar, I see you, I see your struggles, and I want you to know that you are not alone. We are in this battle together. So, to that I say, "Namaste," but I tweak the interpretation slightly to mean, "The divine fight in me salutes the divine fight in you."

I recognize that there is an undying spirit within you. I honor the part of you that won't quit, the part that battles hard despite what the doctors say, and the part that's doing your very best to live your greatest life. I see the light and strength in you because the same light and strength exists within me. And to that I say, "Namaste, my fellow yogi."

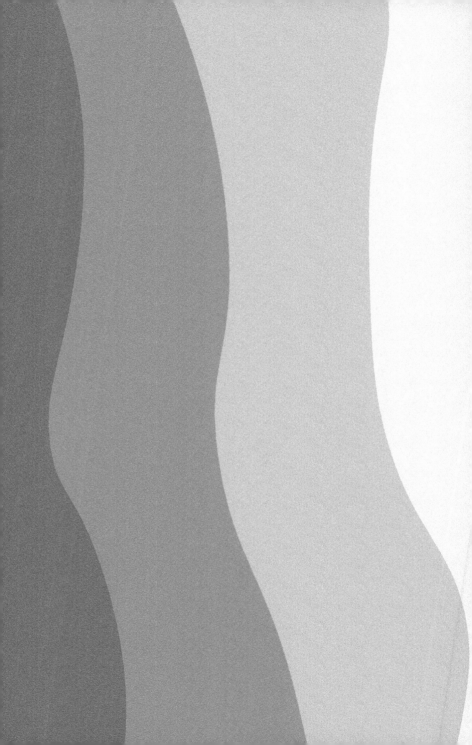

QUICK GUIDE
Daily Practice

Use this quick guide to help you remember the steps to establish a daily practice. But don't forget, you're allowed to make your own rules, so if these don't work for you, find the things that do!

Breathe: Take a slow deep breath, hold it in, then exhale. Repeat as many times as necessary.

Move: Wiggle your toes, go for a walk, practice a few poses. Every day do what feels good for you.

Close Your Eyes: Look inward to let the outside world disappear. Don't fret about the past or worry about the future.

Meditate: Find a single point of focus and draw your attention to it for as long as you can.

Set an Intention: Create a purpose for your day that gives you motivation to keep moving forward. Write it down or say it to yourself.

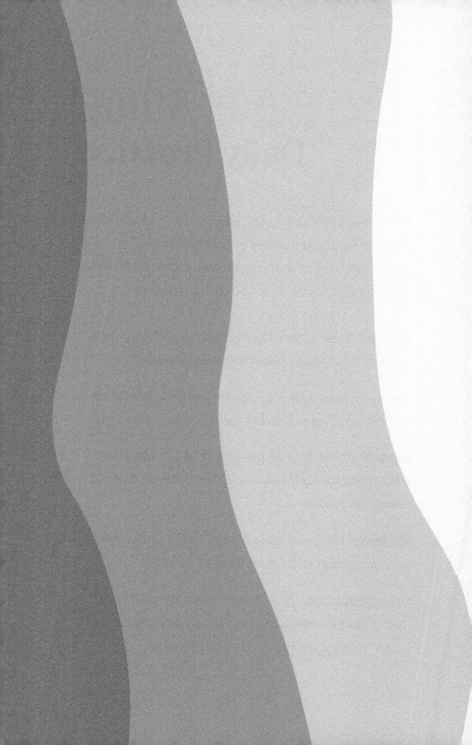

REFERENCE LIBRARY
Poses and Philosophies

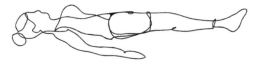

Savasana: Be Here Now

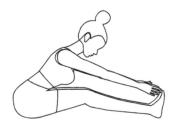

Forward Fold: Give Yourself Props

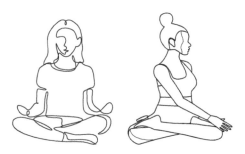

Easy Pose: Slow Down
and Embrace the Beginner Within

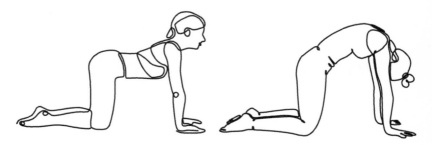

Cat/Cow: Practice makes life

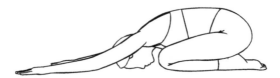

Child's Pose: Listen to Your Body

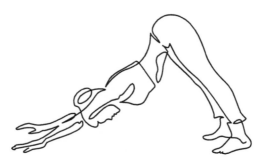

Down Dog: Close Your Eyes

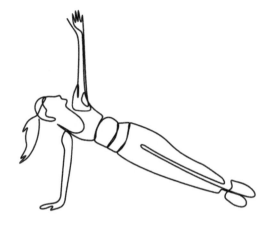

Side Plank: Stop Comparing Yourself to Others

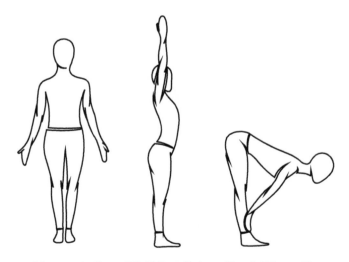

Mountain Pose/Half Sun Salute: Don't Worry Be

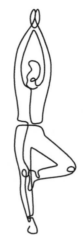

Tree: You Are Not Alone

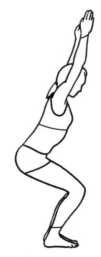

Chair: Just Say No

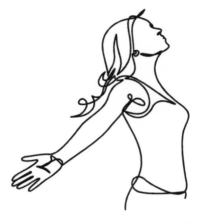

Be Free: Stop Playing by the Rules

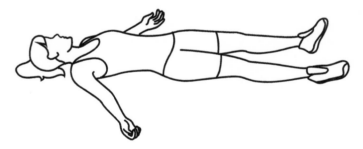

Savasana: Surrender to What Is

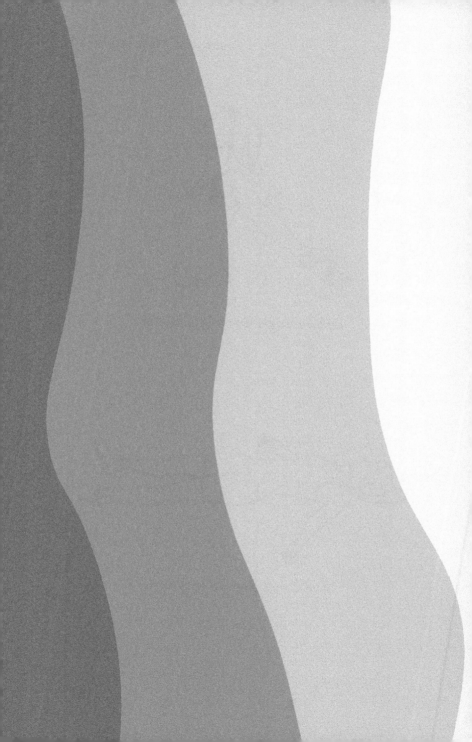

ACKNOWLEDGEMENTS

Having a community to support you when you're dealing with chronic illness is essential. The same is true when writing a book.

Thank you to my family for your never-ending support. Mom, Dad, Cassie, you guys have always been my rock when it comes to dealing with all of my health issues. You let me cry and laugh through every bit of it without judgement. But more than that you never let me give up on my writing, especially this book.

Thank you, Greg, for being my partner through it all.

Many, many thanks to my fellow chronic illness community on social media. I would be lost if I couldn't scroll through Instagram. Seeing a familiar or a new face, a story, or a word of encouragement or commiseration, helps me get through each day. We need each other and I'm so glad a place exists for us to connect from the comfort of our beds!

To my yoga teachers, Alexandria Crow and James Brown, who taught me everything I needed to know. To Nicole Sciacca for suggesting I try my hand at teaching in the first place and giving me a yoga home. Oh, Hustle and Flow, how I miss you!

Thank you to my editors who helped shape this book into a better version than it began. Aleks Mendel thank you for pushing me to dig deeper. Deri Reed you're truly the best. You always get my voice and know how to make it shine.

To the guys at Heads of State, Dustin Summers, Jason Kernevich, and Brandon Wherley, your creativity and attention to detail always help a book make a great first impression. To the Book Designers, Alan Dino Hebel and Ian Koviak, for pulling this whole thing together into a book I'm proud to share with the world.

And finally, thank you to all my students and readers. You are the reason I keep wanting to share my story.

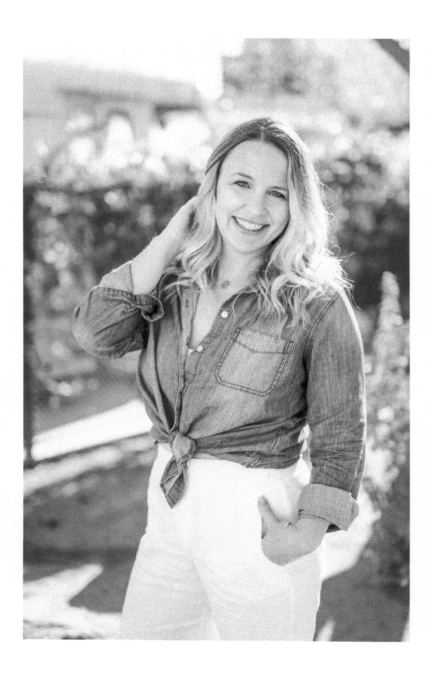

ABOUT THE AUTHOR

Cory Martin is the author of a variety of books including the bestselling *Yoga for Beginners* and the award-winning *Love Sick*, which chronicles her life with multiple sclerosis. She is a chronic illness expert for Verywell Health and her writing has been featured on CNN, HuffPost, Everyday Health, Psychology Today, and more. As a 500-hour certified yoga instructor she's taught at studios across Los Angeles and is the writer behind the documentary *Titans of Yoga*.

To learn more chronic illness survival tips, yoga philosophies and poses, follow Cory on:

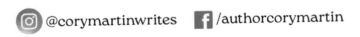 @corymartinwrites /authorcorymartin

Or visit her website:
www.corymartinwrites.com

Lightning Source UK Ltd.
Milton Keynes UK
UKHW011027110122
396962UK00003B/242